THE BRIDGE

THE BRIDGE

MAKING A DIFFERENCE ON A PATIENT'S WORST DAY:
FOR THE PHYSICIAN ASSISTANT AND EMERGENCY
NURSE PRACTITIONER SEEKING TO IMPROVE
PATIENT EXPERIENCE OF CARE

Gary Josephsen MD

ISBN: 0692810005
ISBN 13: 9780692810002

To my wife:
You are everything to me, and without you I'm lost.

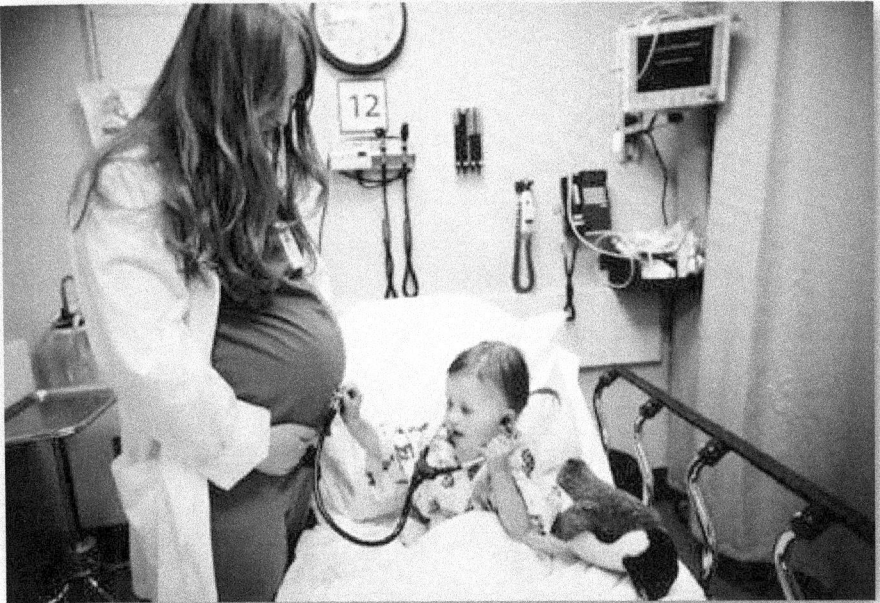

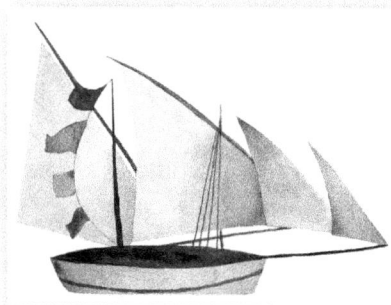

INTRODUCTION

VALUE IN EMERGENCY MEDICINE

Conveyed value = Provider work × Patient perceptions

A s an ED provider, the quality of your care is easy enough for you to see. You've put in the work, during training and throughout your busy shift, to provide quality care for your patient. When you need to go the extra mile, you will, and you'll feel pride in the value you create. But the reason it's easy for you to see that value is because you are an expert. Your patient usually is not, at least when it comes to emergency medicine. So how do we convey to our patients the value of our care? What providers find is that true, unassailable value can go unrecognized in the ED. Because of negative perceptions, your hard work can go unnoticed. There is a disconnect between the quality of care and the experience of care. Let's take a look from the providers' point of view.

Providers John and Kate each graduated from the same program and began careers in emergency medicine. Both had substantial student loan debt and needed to do well in their first job. They felt well prepared at graduation. But each was surprised by how much medicine they still needed to learn.

Emergency medicine is stressful. The pace is frenetic, the atmosphere chaotic, and there is a constant stream of different medical problems. Patients often come in with what seems like a straightforward diagnosis before new information radically changes the picture. Some patients become unstable and die before a diagnosis can be made, slipping away like sand through our fingers. For new providers like John and Kate, it can feel overwhelming.

John responded to the stress by studying ruthlessly to learn the details of clinical emergency medicine. He pored over books, journals, and lectures to absorb the information. He mastered the physical exam and learned which clinical features were most important. With this information, he could make a diagnosis more quickly by recognizing the patterns. With practice, he was also able to make decisions faster. Once he got his feet under him, he could relax, and this freed up his working memory so he could think more creatively. His confidence grew, and the work became less stressful for him.

Kate took the same approach. She studied, read, listened, and made clinical curiosity a daily habit, just like John. But she did something else as well.

Kate had survived a childhood illness that forced her to spend a fair amount of time in the ED as a patient herself. This changed how she learned, allowing her to draw from real-life experience. She went beyond just the science and learned the art of conveying value. She sought to see how her patients viewed her care, not in a superficial way but with ownership and conviction. When someone asked her why patient experience mattered to her, she couldn't think of a good answer, but she was certain that it did.

As they progressed through the early years of their careers, both John and Kate did well. They found emergency medicine practice groups where they fit in well. Their clinical competence outpaced the stress of their new jobs, which they settled into.

But then something happened.

John found that, at times, he felt dread while driving to work. He felt unease whenever his director, who supervised the physician assistants, would sit next to him, wondering whether he might start another discussion about a patient who complained about John's care. He also felt frustrated when, on occasion, his patients asked for a different provider or told him they did not plan to follow his advice. Few patients seemed grateful. Stress once again took hold, and John felt burned out, even though he had just started his career.

Kate was having a different experience. She had started out a little behind John on the medical aspects of the job, but quickly caught up. Her patients were not much different from John's, and the two of them worked in the same ED. But Kate often stayed late at work. She was absorbed in her work and would lose track of time, sometimes staying late. This wasn't because she couldn't keep up, but because she wanted to stay. Her patients were grateful so often that she stopped noticing it, and nurses looked forward to her shifts because the department seemed calmer when she worked. Few of her patients left angry or frustrated. It was very different from John's day-to-day experience.

John and Kate practiced virtually identical medicine, but with very different outcomes. John eventually quit and changed careers altogether. His experience had left him with a bitter taste in his mouth and massive student loans to pay off. Kate learned a different approach.

In this book you will learn what she does differently. It will lower your malpractice risk, increase your longevity, and help you enjoy your days in the ED even more. You will see that managing patient perceptions is less about who you are and more about the environment you create in your practice. It's important to know which parts of the encounter matter the most and why so that you, knowing how perceptions magnify the value of your work, won't need to go through the pain that John went through.

Kate did not need to go through the pain that John experienced because her patient care ended with the encounter. She didn't need to spend time troubleshooting or discussing patient complaints with her director. In fact, although she had a few patient complaints and, once in a while, some angry patients, most were grateful. This left her feeling appreciated and that she was on the right course in life. She was fulfilling her purpose.

Kate's patients had very positive perceptions of her care. The work that she put in was magnified by those positive perceptions. These patients left the ED feeling they had received something of value.

At some point, we choose which path to take. Kate had survived a childhood illness, which gave her a unique perspective that helped her interact with patients. John worked just as hard at learning medicine, but the daily grind was harder on him because he lacked the positive interactions and appreciation that sustained Kate. The difference was not the amount of work these providers put in, but rather their patients' perception of that work. Kate's work conveyed value to her patients, while John's was left open to interpretation.

———

Bridge of trust

Providers often find out too late that they have lost rapport. Usually it happens at the end of the visit or afterward. They might find out because a patient becomes angry when he or she is discharged, or later when they file a complaint. During the encounter most patients keep their bad experiences concealed. You'll often have no idea until it's too late. In fact, studies show that most unhappy patients never complain.

When you first sit down at the ED bedside, you and your patient are divided. You stand on one side of a metaphorical cliff, and the patient on the other. When you build rapport it acts as a bridge of trust between you. This bridge is the foundation of your therapeutic relationship. At the conclusion of your encounter you'll ask the patient to accept your diagnosis or reassurance. Then it's simple: if you've built the bridge well, they'll just step across. But if there are gaps, then who can blame them for hesitating? This book is about that bridge and how to build it.

We will go over the details of how to quickly build a strong bridge throughout these pages. But remember, if you have inadequate rapport when it's time to deliver the diagnosis, asking your patients to trust you is like asking them to step into a void. This won't make sense to them, and it will be too late.

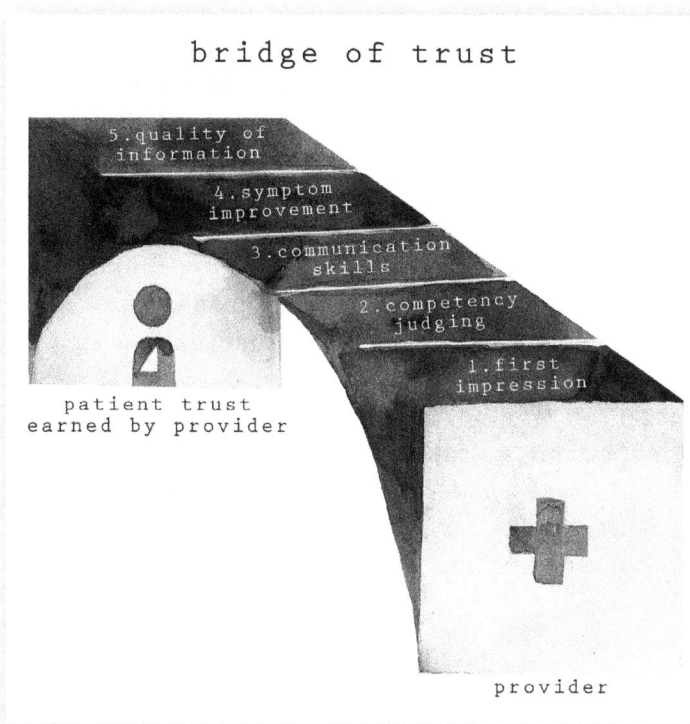

bridge of trust

5.quality of information

4.symptom improvement

3.communication skills

2.competency judging

1.first impression

patient trust earned by provider

provider

Value of this skillset

You have invested part of your life in learning medicine—years lost to learning. As medicine changes, you will need to learn anew what has changed, like new therapies or antibiotic choices. It will take time and energy. The good news is that some skills, like the ones that help shape patient perception, do not change. Learning to convey value in emergency medicine can be hard, but once it's done, it's done. These skills are then applicable to every patient, regardless of the situation. When mastered, they will serve you for life.

When you learn to convey value, your skills act as a fulcrum to help lift your patients' understanding of what you do for them in the ED. It creates more payoff for your efforts.

Much of this payoff comes from increased feelings of satisfaction and control in your work. You will also develop a feeling of increased connectedness to your patients, and be viewed as an asset to your group.

Poor patient perceptions come at a high price. Gerald Hickson, a pediatrician and researcher whom we will revisit later in this book, found that physicians with repeated patient complaints had a higher risk of being named in malpractice lawsuits. This is a glaring reality in practice.

Many lawsuits, whether legitimate or not, begin with a breakdown in communication or fractured trust. Most are not based on poor care, but rather the perception of poor care. Learning to demonstrate the value of your care decreases risk. Malpractice companies know this, supervising physicians know this, and hospital-administration staff know this. They are all invested in your ability to convey value. If gaining expertise in this skill set can prevent even one lawsuit, then it's worth as much as the $3 million cap on your malpractice insurance.

More importantly, patients are more likely to adhere to a treatment plan when providers build a therapeutic partnership with their patients. Adherence to the plan makes them healthier, which improves their life.

Providers who effectively communicate with their patients have a calming effect on their departments, and this is not lost on their colleagues. They are recognized as leaders in their group. When people see excellence in one area, it's easy to see it in other areas as well.

The converse is also true.

When a provider's day is filled with poor interactions, it creates a negative work environment with unpredictable stress. As stress goes, unpredictable stress is worse than predictable stress. These providers often feel burned out after their shifts, and it can be unpleasant to work with them. The negative feelings spill over. Everyone in the department feels on edge—nurses, techs, clerks, and other providers. Providers who underestimate the importance of patient perceptions do so at their peril. When patients don't see the value of your work, your work life becomes harder.

Emotional investment in your work will inoculate you against burnout. Highly skilled providers feel more engaged and less stressed. This protects them when times get rough.

It's not easy. There is emotional labor involved in mastering interpersonal skills. Disciplining oneself to implement the techniques every day, every hour, with every patient, is hard. But again, the skills won't change, they apply to every patient, and they give providers job control. Competency in managing patient perceptions is rewarded with greater job security and satisfaction.

As providers we take an oath to do no harm and to continually develop our medical knowledge. We pledge ourselves to lifelong learning. Some might ask, why not improve patient care simply by mastery of medicine? Why not just learn more medicine and convey value by delivering better care? In fact, this book assumes you will, but that alone is not enough. Excellent care isn't always self-evident. Patient perception is complex.

barriers to connection

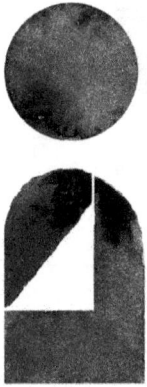

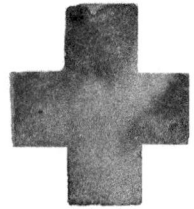

-different cultures
-cognitive biases
-structure of the
 ED encounter

There is often a disconnect between the quality of the care and a patient's experience. At times, you will reenter the room and find a rift

regression to the mean fallacy

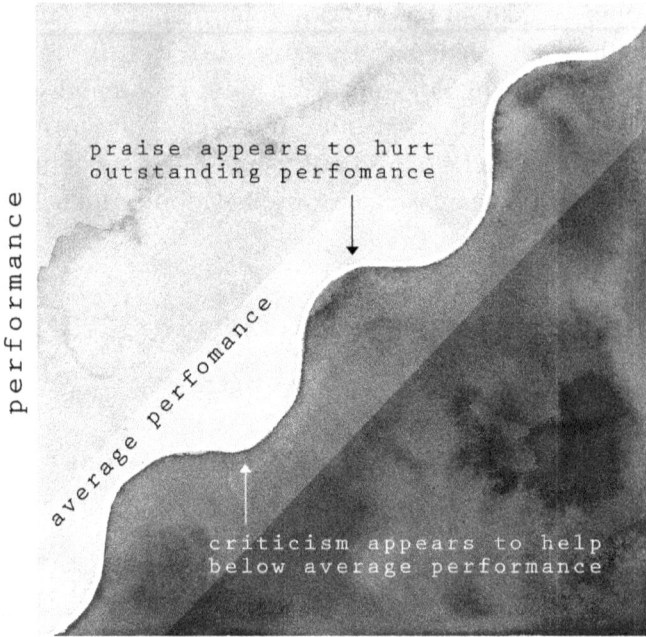

praise appears to hurt
outstanding perfomance

performance

average perfomance

criticism appears to help
below average performance

evaluations during training

*actual variation in performance
is due largely to chance

between you and the patient. They did not appreciate the work you did. In truth, you did well and went the extra mile for them, but it has gone unrecognized. Such occasions are found throughout emergency medicine, which lags behind primary care in Gallup polls measuring patient satisfaction, despite its convenience and the cutting-edge technology it employs.

Why is there a disconnect? Why would a patient feel unsatisfied despite receiving an adequate standard of care? There are three main reasons:

1. Patients and providers have fundamentally **different cultures**, with different priorities and views of illness.
2. **Cognitive biases,** known as heuristics, influence our view of the world. They are to our cognitive systems what optical illusions are to our visual system, and they sometimes blind our perception.
3. The ED encounter **structure** strains interpersonal interactions already hindered by these biases.

Regression to the mean fallacy: Why is managing patient perception hard to learn?

Learning to manage patient perception can be difficult. This is because it is complex, and learning a complex new task requires constant feedback to the learner. Unfortunately, feedback is usually erratic and unreliable. And erratic feedback can make what we do seem effective even when it isn't working.

Psychologists Amos Tversky and Daniel Kahneman, interested in fighter-pilot training, found that most fighter-pilot instructors had very strong opinions about training their pilots. These instructors had undergone similar training and had been teaching complex combat aviation for years. They thought they knew the best way to learn, but they were wrong.

The flight instructors had been fooled by a cognitive bias called the regression to the mean fallacy, which led them to see patterns that weren't really there.

They strongly preferred negative feedback over positive feedback. These teachers believed that positive feedback was not effective because it did not motivate the younger pilots to improve.

Kahneman and Tversky found that fighter-pilot maneuvers were complex and difficult to master. When a student performed at an above-average level, this was usually followed by a more average, and therefore worse, performance.

Although the students were getting better over time, average performances were more common than outliers. Poorer performances were also generally followed by more average performances, but because average performance was better than the poor, it looked like improvement.

The overall trend was improvement, but each flight performance was somewhat random: good flight, average flight, poor flight, average flight. Because fighter-pilot exercises are complicated, like medical encounters, they are hard to evaluate. This did not stop their instructors from seeing patterns, even when the patterns were an illusion. Statistical analysis showed variation to be largely random. The patterns weren't real.

When a student was reprimanded for a bad performance and then did better (returning to a more average performance), the instructors believed their negative feedback had worked. Negative feedback seemed to be followed by improvement, even though, statistically, variation was random.

Positive feedback seemed to hurt because whenever someone did well, then was praised for it, the next performance was merely average. The pattern seen by the instructors fit their intuition about how to train pilots, so they accepted it without question.

In their paper,[2] Tversky and Kahneman argued that the instructors were biased. They saw their feedback as affecting performance when, in fact, it hadn't. Performance over time tended toward average. We see this in other areas too. Good days tend to be followed by average days, great performances by mediocre ones, and husbands of brilliant women tend to be dull compared to their spouses. (Just ask my wife.)

In the ED, we have a similar bias. Most patients have average experiences and an average level of contentment with their care (ambivalence). Most patients who suffer through bad experiences have a tendency not to complain. The frequency of bad interactions is low and erratic. In a perfect world, we would know every time the patient felt unsatisfied, and the reason. But we don't. For this reason, providers have huge blind spots when it comes to how they are perceived. There is little helpful feedback.

Providers who receive negative feedback get it in clusters. Sometimes complaints will come to you all at once, other times they will sporadically trickle in—all because of randomness. Because it is mostly random, the feedback you receive is unlikely to be helpful. Remember that most

2 Daniel Kahneman and Amos Tversky, "On the Psychology of Prediction," *Psychological Review* 80 (1973): 237–57.

patients don't complain. When you change one detail of your care and the complaints go away, you might assume the problem is fixed, even when it isn't. Getting accurate feedback in real time is impossible.

Your supervisors, like the fighter-pilot instructors, will also see patterns where there are none. You'll get lots of negative feedback that is not helpful.

Patient-satisfaction experts and your supervisors will have a list of extra things to do or say to help improve patient experience, but in a complex, fast-paced ED there isn't enough time with each patient. This book is a distillation of the most important moments in an ED encounter. It's a practical approach. Improving patient experience of care involves both tactics and strategy. Tactics means doing things right, like the helpful suggestions from experts about MORE things to do during the encounter. But more is not always better, and you will need to be selective about which parts of the encounter to modify. This is where strategy comes in. You will need to decide which techniques will be high yield. You need to do things right, but you also need to do the right things.

Anatomy of the book

Part 1, Making a Difference on Their Worst Day, begins with an anthropologist, Irwin Press, who began studying folk healers in rural Latin America. His perspective showed him things unseen by physicians in the modern world. He recognized the disconnect between quality of care and experience of care. He went from being an outsider, rejected by the medical community, to a primary authority on patient satisfaction in emergency medicine. We will explore, based on the lessons learned by Press, different strategies for closing the gap between patient and provider. Next, we will explore what cognitive science can teach us about problems with our perceptions. We will see that, because of our evolution in tribes, we are sometimes maladapted to our modern environment. Using this insight, it becomes clear that some moments in the ED carry more weight than others when it comes to patient perception. These moments act like fulcrums to convey to patients the value their provider delivers.

Part 2, The Checklist, builds a checklist to change the structure of the ED encounter. It continues by drawing on the insights from Press and cognitive science to collect the best strategies for conveying value. Instead of continually adding extra steps to an already busy ED visit, part II carves a list of key nonmedical needs, as well as steps to meet those needs with every patient. We will revisit John and Kate as they continue in their careers.

Part 3, The Tribe, recognizes the holistic nature of patients' experience in the ED. It introduces the ship model of practice, where dysfunctional behavior can be like holes in the hull, and your medical team, the ship's crew. Many providers follow tactics to optimize their patients' experience, only to fail because of team dysfunction or other disruptive behavior. In this section, we meet Gerald Hickson, who created a system in his community to give patients a voice and to hold physicians accountable. We see how it helped to dramatically lower the frequency of malpractice lawsuits, and we'll learn why Hickson believes modern medical professionalism must go beyond basic medical competency. After this, we will discuss practical aspects of conveying value to each member of our medical team: our nurses, supervising physicians, and consultants. Then, we will learn advanced techniques for bridging gaps in patient perception, such as customer-service rescue.

It's frustrating not to have your efforts appreciated. Many patients don't know it, but in the emergency department you, the provider, are at a huge disadvantage. You have limited time and limited information, but are still accountable for accurately diagnosing your patients' problems quickly. With the pressure on, you work hard and manage to knock it out of the park. A diagnosis made, a life saved. Finding out that a patient is still not happy feels like a betrayal. How can someone for whom so much has been done be so ungrateful? In fact, most of these patients are not habitually ungrateful. They are just normal people who have had an experience they didn't appreciate. It is possible for patients to have a good outcome, where the provider saved their life, and still feel genuinely unsatisfied. It happens every day, but it doesn't have to.

Each day, we make small decisions that direct our life: small changes that have significant long-term impact. At the time, we don't appreciate how these choices will impact our lives, but they do. They impact our lives and the lives of those around us. My hope is that this book will set a course that will benefit both you and your patients. Remember that what you do matters, but how you do it matters, too.

PART 1: MAKING A DIFFERENCE ON THEIR WORST DAY

CHAPTER 1

PATIENT PERCEPTION IN THE EMERGENCY DEPARTMENT

There are two fundamental ways of looking at the world. One popular philosophy is that the world exists as it is: trees are green, sugar is sweet, and coffee is bitter. In this view, everything we see or touch has a quality that everyone else would know if they saw or touched it. There is no room for interpretation.

The other view is that everything is open to interpretation. We might agree that coffee is bitter, but each of us experiences the taste of coffee in a slightly different way. Some may taste quiet hazelnut notes, others a touch of wheat. We agree that the traffic light is red and that we must stop, but is your red the same as my red? In this view, each person's perspective is unique.

We know from a strictly scientific point of view that the second philosophy is the truth. Each person grows from a baby and has unique equipment—eyes, ears, and intellect—that they use to view the world. The tricky thing is that it's easy to take this for granted. We forget this subtle truth. If you asked for a summary of this book in one sentence, it would be this: to see what someone else sees, you have to look through their eyes.

The view from inside a hospital gown

If reasonable people should be content with quality care, then why is patient satisfaction so hard to achieve?

Imagine a woman named Joy, a mother of two and a college-educated homemaker, coming to the ED. She had chest pain.

At first she waited for it to go away, not sure if it was dangerous. After the pain continued, she decided to come in and get checked. Joy has had few ED visits in her life. She is pretty healthy and active, and has certain subconscious expectations about what she wants from her ED visit.

First on the list is a competent provider. Joy has heard horror stories about patients hurt by bad doctors. She'd naturally like to have the most skilled provider possible but, if not available, at least someone who is competent and unlikely to maim her.

She is also hoping that, when she meets the provider, they will know why she is having chest pain. What is causing it? How do you make it go away so she can feel normal again? She has things to get done. People depend on her, and she needs to get back to her life. Feeling better is also near the top of the list, and if this is a heart attack, she wants to have it fixed. She hopes for a cure and for relief from her symptoms.

After that short list of top priorities there are other things that would be nice. For example, she doesn't want to sit in the waiting room and maybe catch the flu while waiting her turn. She understands the ED experience only moves so fast. It's not like she thinks of health care as a convenience, but no reasonable person wants to sit all day in the waiting room.

Cost is also a concern. The visit should be relatively affordable, maybe even frugal, if it doesn't sacrifice quality; just like any other part of her life. Money doesn't grow on trees and insurance companies have a tendency to not pay the whole bill.

It occurs to Joy as she sits in the busy waiting room that her chest pain is much better. It would really sting if this was a false alarm that ended up massively disrupting her life, with expensive hospital bills and maybe even a stay in the hospital for tests.

Joy does not want to waste her time. She thought hard about whether to come to the ED and doesn't want to have made an expensive mistake.

There are also fears sitting in the back of Joy's mind. What if she is misdiagnosed or has a reaction to one of the medicines? What if she has a bad reaction and feels worse than when she came in? She also worries that she might be too young to have a heart attack. Will the nurses think she is crazy?

What if she forgets some of her symptoms and doesn't tell the provider? And what if this leads to an incorrect diagnosis? Or no diagnosis at all? What if there is a mistake and the wrong treatment is given? She could be harmed by not telling them all the information. She could be harmed if they blow off an important detail she does mention.

A major source of unease is the lack of familiarity Joy has with the whole process. She doesn't know where to go or what will happen next. It's unclear when she will pay or what the final bill will be. She has no information about the provider, and there is no way for her to check how good they are on the Internet because medicine is not her area of expertise, and the hospital's Wi-Fi is really slow.

The weight on the shoulders of an ED provider

Contrast this to the more familiar perspective of John, the ED provider. When he arrives at work, he genuinely hopes he'll have a chance to improve someone's health or maybe even save their life. He is altruistic. He wants to relieve suffering and make a diagnosis, or at least rule-out emergencies.

Like most providers, he considers cost-effective care important, although the practical aspects of containing cost are sometimes difficult to identify.

He wants to be thorough and avoid mistakes. He wants to avoid over-testing and anything that may expose the patient to unnecessary risks. His goals are to detect emergencies on time to intervene, to protect his patients' well-being, and to avoid waste and inefficiency, so he can get things done in a reasonable amount of time.

Perhaps he can see all the patients in the lobby before the next provider is scheduled to start, so they will have a clean slate. That would be great.

To accomplish this, he often has to focus on the details of the department. Was the blood sent to the lab? When will it be back? Why is x-ray backed up? Are we really out of urine cups? Troubleshooting the complexities of the ED can give him a myopic viewpoint. With the pressures of the ED, he is somewhat blinded to the perspectives of his colleagues and patients. There is a lot on his mind while he works.

———

As Joy gets checked in, she's relieved to have a warm, kind nurse who treats her with respect. It feels like Joy has known this woman for a long time. Even though they just met, they have made a connection. While Joy is hesitant to ask too many questions for fear that she might appear needy, she is relieved to have this nurse.

The nurse asks her questions about why she came in, the details of her chest pain, her medical history, etc. Some of the questions seem irrelevant to Joy. She tries to tell the nurse the specifics about her pain, worried she might forget an important detail. The nurse redirects her to get through the list of questions on the computer.

After Joy disrobes, she is hooked up to a machine. A tech tears off her ECG and walks out of the room with it. She is given a blanket that feels nice and warm, and then she is left alone. The blood pressure cuff squeezes her arm until it feels like it cuts off her blood. She waits; the pain seems better. Maybe she should have stayed home? She shakes her head.

———

Modern medicine and disconnection

There are differences in perspective between the patient and the provider. Some of the differences come from the different roles, but some are unique to our modern emergency departments.

Humans evolved in tribes. Prior to modern medicine, folk healers were the primary means to getting well. In the history of the world, human beings have existed for only the blink of an eye, preceded by thousands of years of uneventful geological time. In the same way, modern medicine has come only recently, another blink of the eye in the long history of human healing.

Our evolution in tribes has selected a brain system highly efficient for life in small groups. We are adept at judging intentions, deciding quickly who might be a threat or an ally. This system hasn't had time to evolve and adapt to our modern environment, or to the technical revolution of medicine. The result is a mind that is adept at making flash judgments about who we want in our tribes, but poor at judging the competency of medical providers.

As providers, we want our patients to feel better, but we are also trained to rely on firm scientific endpoints. We want the blood pressure to come down to normal, for the tachycardia to resolve, and we are fixated on the patient's white blood cell count. For us, these objective measures add scientific rigor to our investigation of the patient's symptoms and give us a sense of confidence in our evaluation.

As patients—and we will all be patients at some point—our endpoints are more in line with human evolutionary origins: we want to feel better. We also want to be able to tell our story completely. There is catharsis and relief in knowing that your provider understands all the details of your illness. After patients tell their story, they can relax. Otherwise, patients may feel an uncomfortable burden from holding all the details of their story in their working memory, unable to let it rest. After clearing the working memory of all the details, and knowing those details will not be lost, even painful conditions can become easier to bear.

―――

Joy meets her provider, John. They do not connect. She begins telling him her story but does not get to finish because John is called out during their brief meeting. He seems young and abrupt. It doesn't seem as if he hears everything she says. His questions are things she has already covered with the nurse. Frankly, he doesn't seem like a very good provider. John tells her the tests will be back soon, asks her to rate her pain, and then disappears.

―――

The disconnect between quality-care delivery and patient experience comes from different perspectives between patients and providers. Some of these differences come simply from the different priorities held by each. Others stem from our ancient origins. Our minds are better evolved for the kind of encounter we might have with a tribal folk healer than with a fast-paced and technically modern ED. The differences in perspective serve as a divide between patients and providers, and it's difficult to connect across the divide.

Joy has no medical training. Her priorities and expectations are very different from those of her provider. This difference in viewpoint separates the two from forming a therapeutic partnership.

———

Now I'd like to let you in on a secret: I'm John. My struggles with patient interaction led to pain early in my career. I could feel the stress, and when I tried to change my habits, things seemed to work for a while, but then more complaints would add up. I believed in the importance of satisfaction, and in the value of my patients' perceptions, but I just couldn't make things work.

Because of this I chose to seek out an expert and found several good mentors. First I'd like to tell you about a man whose name is synonymous with patient satisfaction in the Emergency Department: Irwin Press, co-founder of Press Ganey, a company specializing in ED patient-satisfaction surveys.

The first widely used measure of ED patient satisfaction was the Press Ganey survey. In fact, many experienced providers get a little queasy when they hear the phrase "Press Ganey Score." This became the tool that was used to compare providers and hospitals, and even served to provide feedback used to evaluate providers who were struggling to convey value. Press, who published his experience in a book called *Patient Satisfaction*, agreed to meet me for dinner in Chicago on a warm summer evening.

CHAPTER 2

IRWIN PRESS AND THE WITCH DOCTORS

To find answers, I arrive in Chicago and head downtown to meet Irwin Press. The truth is I'm nervous. He is, I expect, a polished expert. I am, secretly, a doctor who doesn't have good Press-Ganey scores. I don't plan to bring that up. At this point, I've read his book and tried, with limited success, to put its recommendations into practice. I often feel like I'm doing it wrong, just like when I waited tables as a high-school student. Back then, someone once asked me for two pieces of bread after I brought them just one. I broke it into two halves, and then asked if they'd like more pieces. I probably won't bring that up with Press either.

When we meet face to face, I'm surprised to find that he is shorter than I, silver haired, and with eyes that wrinkle warmly around the edges when he smiles. He wears a jacket that makes him look like a college professor. I find out that's because he was a professor, at Notre Dame, where he taught anthropology. He is no longer at Press-Ganey.

My expectations of Dr. Press, who is not a medical doctor, could not have been more wrong. Although he's articulate, he is also very informal. He tells jokes, old jokes. He is gracious and tells me his story. He never intended to create a company, let alone survey ED patients, he said. He was an anthropologist, only interested in people.

Medical acculturation in rural Latin America

The son of immigrant parents, Press grew up in Andersonville, a Swedish neighborhood on the north side of Chicago. As a child in an immigrant community, he had experiences that affected the way he approached his work, much like Kate, the provider who spent many days in the ED herself as a child. His passion became anthropology, the study of norms and values in societies, but his background interest in immigrant groups created a fascination with the process of acculturation, which is how groups adopt the social patterns of other groups.

Culturally diverse groups sometimes relocate from the countryside to an urban area, like Chicago or Delhi. Initially they organize in groups within their original ethnicities, but then people begin to adopt the traits of other cultures, and they blend. Press explained this to me as we sat down to dinner at a Greek restaurant in a part of the city which, he says, has become regentrified. This place has great food, he adds, and we order wine as he begins:

> *[Anthropology] opened the world to me. And it helped me to explain, or I thought that I could explain, why people behaved the way they do. And it also opens your eyes when you realize you're not alone, and that there are others out there who have a very different perspective, who have a worldview that…that's based on completely different concepts than you. You can either do it yourself at that point and say "the hell with them, I don't even care if they're wrong, whatever it is," or "Oh my God, I'm not the only person here."*

He began his studies observing indigenous people in Mexico who were in contact with modern cities, and would later continue this work in Bogotá, Colombia. In those places, similar to immigrants in Chicago, natives moved to urban areas and came into contact with other cultures. This began the process of acculturation, taking on some social practices while avoiding other changes. Press was primarily interested in which practices they would adopt and why.

> *[I] did my fieldwork in Yucatán, Mexico. A village called Pustunich that was about 2 miles outside of Ticul, right in the center, about an hour, two hours south of Mérida…what I had there was a village that was confronting change, yet at the same time, maintaining its integrity.*

[Later, in Bogotá,] I wanted to continue to study the process of culture change. How do people change? And in the process, what do they do with old behaviors as new behaviors replace them? So, I decided to focus on health care, and look at immigrants who came into Bogotá, and look at their health care. Under what circumstances do they go to doctors?

Press's story wasn't starting out as I had expected. I anticipated hearing about patients in the ED, and surveys. Instead we were talking about native people in Colombia. Maybe it was because I had also worked in Bogotá and remembered it being extremely dangerous and gritty. The Guerilla rebels had destroyed large parts of the city, and young boys guarded buildings with automatic weapons. Gunfire broke the silence at night, and twice large groups of people were massacred outside the city. What I remembered was fear. Press didn't mention the dangerous parts at all. Instead he told me that he wasn't really interested in medical practices. He was interested in how immigrants undergo acculturation, and how social norms drive their choice of physician.

At that time in Bogotá, Press had discovered native groups who had relocated to the city, where they had access to modern medicine. He found that both there and in rural Mexico, some people would prefer to see traditional folk healers instead of modern physicians. He also found some folk healers who had relocated to the city and set up shop there. He called these the Urban Curaderos, but would sometimes refer to folk healers as witch doctors, a term that held no negative connotations for him.

So anyway, there I was in Bogotá. I was going to the big clinic...observing patients, observing doctors work with patients, and I was observing witch doctors work with the patients. So I was interested in seeing under what circumstances people use [folk medicine] and under what circumstances they use their clinic.

He found this very interesting because it was a clear example of acculturation that could be observed across different cultural melting pots. Why would people choose folk medicine over modern medicine? Did modern medicine not seem better? Were there barriers to accessing health care? What could people possibly get from a witch doctor that they couldn't get from a "real" doctor? A lot, it turns out.

Closed and open models of illness

Here Press touched an idea that would change his life. He saw that culture was not limited to natives and city dwellers. Modern physicians and their modern patients had differences so contrasting that they were like the cultural differences between different ethnic groups, which sometimes cause conflict or misunderstandings.

This was true even if the physician and patient shared the same ethnicity. Their beliefs were still so different that it was as though they were from different cultures.

Press characterized the main cultural difference between patient and physician as open versus closed models of illness. He called these explanatory models.

To a patient, Press might assert, his or her illness, life circumstances, stress level, and recent experience may all be interconnected. He would call this an open model of illness: the possibility for connections between illness and other parts of life. A closed model of illness would exclude other connections as irrelevant and unscientific. Koch's Postulates, the basis for the germ theory of disease, is a good example of a closed model of illness:

1. **The microorganism must be found in abundance in all organisms suffering from the disease, but should not be found in healthy organisms.**
2. **The microorganism must be isolated from a diseased organism and grown in pure culture.**
3. **The cultured microorganism should cause disease when introduced into a healthy organism.**
4. **The microorganism must be reisolated from the inoculated, diseased experimental host and identified as being identical to the original specific causative agent.**

This is the skeptical and deductive scientific method. It is rigorous and doesn't consider outside influences. Influenza causes the flu, nothing more.

Press explained his observations:

> *I would interview patients at the witch doctor's office, and patients in the [modern] clinic, and I would ask them in each case, what's bothering you? So what is it? One of the things that I got in the witch doctor's office was, they would always typically say, there was a couple of symptoms that were social or emotional. For example, a patient would say something like, "I have this pain in my belly and it's just kind of been moving up into my throat area, and my business has not been so good lately." To the witch doctor, it's all part of a syndrome, maybe witchcraft, you got an enemy. At the clinic, they would completely dismiss the business not doing well, because it's irrelevant.*

Validating complaints

Press also found that patients at the modern clinics interacted differently with the physicians than they did with the folk healers. Specifically, the history they gave changed, and they tended to give additional complaints. He would later refer to these extra complaints as *validating complaints*. Press believed they were given to emphasize legitimacy of an illness and it's severity. He explained:

> *I was saying to the patients, "What's bothering you, what brings you, what else, what else, what else?" until they…ran out of symptoms, I had at least two more symptoms on average at the clinic than at the witch doctors. And the way I figured it, it was simple. Because the witch doctor will take any symptoms you give them, whatever you do, and pay attention to them, but not at a clinic.*

Press interpreted this finding to show that patients at the modern clinic did not feel validated in the same way that they did with their folk healers. He hypothesized that this was because the folk healer would accept their patients' open model of illness without question, whereas the modern physician dismissed extra details as irrelevant. We scoff at the efficacy of folk medicine, but the witch doctors who Press saw were experts in connecting with their patients. And they accepted their patients regardless of the beliefs they brought with them.

> *All of a sudden it became clear. What I suspected was going on with the physician was that the patients would come up with symptoms that might be ignored, so they came up with more symptoms so that at least a couple of them would be focused on, whereas at the witch doctor's office, he'll deal with every [symptom] he was given. In other words, the doctor would ignore what the patient came in with or wasn't relevant to his concept of what may be appropriate.*

Nonmedical need for validation

After some thought I supposed it was not surprising that patients may seek care from traditional folk healers in Latin America. Patients continue to do that today in the United States. The thought of validating an illogical connection of someone's sickness to another voodoo cause, like having an enemy, sounded like charlatanism. But Press wasn't giving me advice. He was telling me his story.

Later, I would realize the relevance. As alluded to in the last chapter, the evolution of medicine has accelerated at an ever-quickening pace. Humanity's existence (two million years) has only been a blink of an eye compared to the age of the earth (4.5 billion years). In the same way, medicine has changed logarithmically during the existence of human illness.

The first documented medical treatments are five thousand years old, written in Sumerian Cuneiform, followed by the Egyptian Ebers Papyrus of three thousand years ago. Apparently ancient Egyptians were the first in recorded history to brush their teeth, but they did so with sand, which eroded the enamel and was therefore probably counterproductive. Hippocrates came about twenty-five hundred years ago at around 460 BC, just before the Han Dynasty in China created scrolls of herbal medicine in AD 200. Syphilis became pandemic in 1495 and was treated (ineffectively) with poisonous mercury. Penicillin wasn't used to treat it until 1943.

In the last fifty years—yes, that's only fifty years—the explosion of technology and medical advancement have accelerated like the geometric curve of a nautilus shell curve. Emergency medicine became a specialty in the late 1960s, and electronic medical records were mandated ten years ago, resulting in a computer in each patient room.

Our bodies and minds, however, have not evolved quite so quickly. We are poorly equipped to thrive in this modern environment. For example, sugar and sitting do not meet the needs of our bodies, which have evolved to hunt for wild game while fasting. Similarly, our minds are not evolved for the modern emergency medicine encounter. Despite efficient technical evaluation, something seems to be missing.

If you took the view of an anthropologist, as Press did, you might reason that something was, and is, driving patients to seek care from folk healers as an alternative to western medicine. There must be some ancient, nonmedical needs that remain unmet. What Press observed was that folk healers met those needs by validating their open model of illness in a way that the modern physicians would not.

Osler's model of detached concern

From the point of view of a trained modern medical provider, it's hard to accept comparisons with native folk medicine. Some might argue that objectivity in medicine has provided the scientific rigor to advance medical science. As a young anthropologist, Press may not have understood (although he may now) the history of objectivity in medicine; what Jodi Halpern, a Berkeley-based expert on clinical empathy, calls *detached concern*.

Still, I felt troubled when I learned about patients who preferred local witch doctors to physicians. All of medical science was finally available to them, yet they weren't interested?

In her book *From Detached Concern to Empathy*, Halpern outlines the history of detached concern in modern medicine:

From the perspective of the early twentieth century, the previous history of medicine was one in which pseudo-scientific practices, such as blood-letting, were ineffective at fighting disease. Physicians found that procedures they once felt hopeful about often did more harm than good. Sympathetic emotions, which were already seen to cause clinical errors seem to have been discredited as old practices.[2]

She traces the origin of objectivity to Rene Descartes, and the belief by Immanuel Kant that emotions, unlike sensory perceptions, are highly subjective and cannot contribute to reason-based decision making:

Emotions are therefore merely subjective impressions and cannot provide any real cognitive value.[3]

She cites Sir William Osler, father of modern medicine, in his 1910 essay, *Aequanimitas.* In it Osler describes the value of equanimity when evaluating a patient's illness. For him, seeing the inner life of a patient had to be done with an objective and detached eye in order to avoid errors or let emotions color one's experience.

While objectivity in decision making may arguably help avoid biases, cognitive science suggests that even objective decision making is riddled with bias. Clinical objectivity has not, at the time of this writing of this book, been shown to improve outcomes. There is little measure of such an objective state, and avoidance of bias may be impossible.

In her book, Halpern is primarily concerned with the therapeutic partnership forged through clinical empathy. She is careful to contrast clinical empathy from standard empathy (which can mean many things). For her, clinical empathy involved curiosity for the patient's own subjective experience, as well as conveying to our patients that they are not alone in their struggle. We are with them.

She goes on to further illustrate the disconnect between the idea of detached concern, often attributed to Osler, and accounts of the reality

---

2 Jodi Hapern, *From Detached Concern to Empathy: Humanizing Medical Practice* (Oxford: Oxford Press, 2001), 21.
3 Ibid.

of Osler's practice style, which was sometimes emotional. He was not strictly objective. Citing him to argue for medical objectivity may be viewed as a contradiction.

It seems that detached concern, like other themes in medicine, is something that we do mainly because it's something we have always done.

Psychoanalysis and countertransference

Freud was also concerned about objectivity, but for another reason. In psychoanalysis, the analyst serves as a sounding board for their patient. On the couch, patients describe their lives, and the psychoanalyst listens, not attempting to provide feedback. This is thought to cause patients to project their subconscious thoughts and emotions onto their therapist, which are then reflected back, like a mirror. This process is called transference. Subconscious thoughts, reflected back to the patient, may then provide therapeutic insight by highlighting and short-circuiting dysfunctional patterns.

Transference of patients' thoughts and emotions can elicit countertransference in the analyst, who at times may experience feelings of hostility toward their patients. Similarly, emergency medicine providers experience negative feelings in their work.

Whether the negative feelings we feel in the ED are due to countertransference or not, they are still part of our experience. The negativity can cloud decision making, create feelings of fatigue, and lead to burnout. ED providers are, no doubt, impacted when exposed to the unbridled emotions of ED patients on the worst day of their lives. Given this negative impact, objectivity or detached concern might be important for professional longevity, in addition to helping make decisions with a clear head.

There are, however, problems with detached concern. It comes at a price.

Detached concern creates distance between the provider and patient, for better or worse. One effect of the distance is the risk of invalidating the significance of a patient's illness. Evolving in tribes, we rely on nonverbal cues to know that our healer understands our situation. If a provider appears objective and unaffected, it relays a nonverbal message: I am not your partner in this, I am objective.

Providers also risk invalidating patients' open model of illness when they focus on details relevant only to the provider's closed model. Take the example from Press: in order to organize my evaluation of your abdominal pain, I first need to know your last menstrual period; then we may continue with the other details. Ignoring details important to patients' open model may, as Press suggests, make them feel invalidated. Patients may respond by adding symptoms to underline the severity of their illness, which Press called validating complaints. For example, the pain was "so intense I passed out," or the pain "made me feel weak and dizzy all over."

The power-distance index

Another distance created by detached concern is what is known as the power-distance index. The power-distance index is the difference in authority between two individuals: pilot and copilot, or provider and patient. In some cultures, patients are evaluated and the physician's recommendations are akin to orders, carried out without question or explanation of medical decision making. Other cultures have a low power-distance index. The provider may need to sell the diagnosis and treatment plan to a patient in order to earn compliance. In the low power-distance example, patients may easily question the authority of the provider and gain additional information without violating social norms.

High power-distance interval relationships lend themselves poorly to open communication. Malcolm Gladwell uses the airline industry to explain cultural differences in power distance in his book *Outliers*.[4] He cited differences in measured power-distance indexes among countries, which roughly correlate with frequency of airline accidents. Gladwell observes that avoiding accidents requires clear crisis communication, and that high power-distance relationships impair open communication.

---

4 Malcolm Gladwell, "The Ethnic Theory of Plane Crashes," in *Outliers: The Story of Success* (New York: Back Bay Books, 2008).

Despite depictions on TV dramas, most EDs aren't often in crisis mode. Neither, however, are most airline flights. Communication gets more strained with stressful situations, and an efficient ED can't afford to let potentially important safety issues go unacknowledged because of high power-distance behavior owing to a tradition of detached concern and scientific objectivity.

Patient-centered approaches focus on their experience, questions, and uncertainty. Most patients are unfamiliar with ED rituals. For an example, take our patient Joy, who didn't understand why she had to repeat her chest-pain history to the triage nurse, the intake nurse, and her provider, John. The value of repeating her story is unclear to her, and the lack of information worsens her stress. Worsening stress strains communication, leaving patients even less informed.

Press believed that folk healers approached healing in a patient-centered way. They validated the patient's illness. And this gave those healers something to offer patients that their modern physician colleagues missed.

CHAPTER 3

RELEVANCE OF MEDICAL ANTHROPOLOGY TO MODERN MEDICINE

P ress would return home from his fieldwork, publish his findings, and share them with his students. From his perspective as the son of immigrant parents, the process of acculturation was intuitive. It fit his experience. But now it was time for Press to recall the maxim that states "to see what someone else sees, you have to look through their eyes." His students, specifically the premed kids, had a different view.

When I got back to Notre Dame I started teaching medical anthropology, looking at different cultures in the world and their healthcare system. And I assumed that pre-med students would find this relevant...So I was teaching medical anthropology...and in the middle of the semester, a student gets up, interrupts me in the middle of my lecture, yells out, "This is all bullshit. This is totally irrelevant for me. I'm going to be a physician practicing in Philadelphia."

That was the key moment in my career. I began to realize, well, I thought, I had a lot of pre-meds in the class and I'd been pretty sure they'd just see a lot of relevance...I wasn't making it clear to them. One reason was that I knew nothing about clinical medicine. So that's when I decided I've got to learn something about [it]...I'm going to be make it relevant to this pre-med.

Press observes modern clinical medicine

To learn more about how this might be relevant to his premed students, Press set up a fellowship where he planned to travel and observe patient care at a large urban training hospital, as an anthropologist. In order to avoid the risk of offending anyone, I will refer to that hospital anonymously as Modern Medicine Memorial. He had the same role as in his previous fieldwork, an outside observer of culture, but instead of observing natives in a village setting, he was in a large urban university hospital. Press would rotate through different departments at the hospital to learn an overview of how clinical medicine is carried out and how this might be relevant to his course on medical anthropology.

Press described his time on the OB Ward at Modern Memorial:

They had a little loudspeaker [for a purple fetal-heart monitor at] 140 beats a minute...I was talking with [a woman in labor] and she had the purple heart monitor and she said, "Look, after you take this off, what are you going to do next to my baby?" And I realized she had no idea of what this was. She didn't realize [the heart monitor] was a passive thing, not an active thing. It wasn't doing anything for her baby or to her baby. They knew nothing. They were given no information.

The need to be informed and validated

Press found that the physicians and patients at Modern Memorial Hospital, like those in his other fieldwork, had radically different perspectives, almost like members of different cultures. Even though he was now in a first-world country at the leading edge of medical science, from the perspective of patient communication there was little difference. He observed the same clash of open and closed models of illness. Keeping patients informed about their care seemed not to be a priority, and these patients had no alternative choice. Moving from Bogotá to Miami should have been a giant step in medical advancement, and indeed it was, but more modern medical care did not seem to translate into improvement when it came to meeting the nonmedical needs of patients. In this respect, they were still behind the folk healers. Medical advancement had not bridged the gap between patient and provider.

The need for respect

Press next told me the story of Cuban immigrant women going into labor in the OB ward.

I noticed that a few women made more noise in labor [so loud] that they knew their husbands heard them…theirs' was a male dominated culture. When they're in labor, [the women] were in charge.

So one day, I saw a husband, just outside the door and a young resident, Anglo resident, with one of the monitors, and she's making all kinds of noise. He actually said, "Look, stop it, it's not that painful, cut it out, stop it." She kept doing it…

The doctor slapped her right on the thigh, hard. He just felt so frustrated. So the point is, he had no idea about the culture of what is going on, nothing.

Sitting at dinner, I was speechless. We sat in silence for a moment. This part of the story was disgraceful and sad. I didn't know what to say, so I just sat and listened.

Press felt that, clearly, something needed to be done, and for him, a big part of the problem was cultural competency. The patient's response to labor was seated in the role of childbirth within their culture, not to mention the fact that labor is actually, well, painful. Press also observed that keeping patients informed was not a priority for residents, who also appeared to lack empathy toward patients. Press felt that feedback needed to be given to the physicians so that they would understand, feel less frustrated, and change the interaction:

Tell the women what's going on, describe and explain what you're doing, pay attention to the local culture, to understand that they're each going to be different, recognizing also that this is a key moment for these women and understand what childbirth means to every culture.

Press continued to explain his concern about the disconnect between the quality of care and the patients' experiences.

I bet if you were to ask any woman you know, "who delivered your baby?" you know what they'll say? They'll give you the doctor's name. Not a one of them will say, "I did." This is the culture we have...I realized also that I had something to offer healthcare...I was getting all kind of insights for things that could be improved in terms of the patient experience. I wasn't yet using the term patient satisfaction [in] 1980.

CHAPTER 4

Patient Satisfaction and Risk Management

P ress gathered his notes and prepared a presentation for the grand rounds at Modern Memorial. He went through his observations and insights about the different cultural nuances creating friction on the ward. He reasoned that if the physicians knew the root of the problem, they would recognize what was happening. Having this insight, they would understand the disconnect between them and their patients. He thought that they would see the world through his eyes and draw the same conclusions he had. I'm sure it will come as no surprise to the reader that this is not what happened.

They did not see things the way he saw them. His words fell stillborn onto the floor.

Press, the outside voice

The response to his observations was doubt. How could an outsider, an Anthropologist PhD without any medical experience, possibly understand the medical process? Remember that the physicians were trained with a philosophy of detached concern, to stand back and view a patient's problem objectively, uninvolved. They viewed what Press called their closed model of illness as medicine itself, beginning, middle, and end. Everything else, including social norms, culture, and the patient's experience of care, was unrelated to their illness. Remember that Press said *this was 1980, and no one was even using the words "patient satisfaction."*

This poor response was discouraging but, at the same time, Press made another connection. Watching women in the midwife ward, he found that they had significantly fewer cesarean sections than in the OB ward. He also felt that these women were treated better. Midwives have, after all, descended from a tradition of folk medicine.

Press made another observation which, like his previous ideas, would first be ignored and then prove to change the course of medical practice for the next fifty years:

> *[I]n the back of my mind was this idea, like you said, the patients have a better experience, personal experience in the hospital, they're less likely [to sue] if something happened. So I look through the closed [malpractice] claims and I realize that 50% of them are unclear. There was no clear injury [to the patient].*

What Press meant was that when malpractice lawsuits are filed, there has to be some form of damage. Either the patient is hurt or gets sicker because the physician fails to do what's needed to be done. Malpractice lawsuits are, presumably, initiated by malpractice; failure to provide basic medical care. But Press found that in many of these suits, there was no clear bad outcome. Instead they began as personal vendetta against a physician who a patient thought was dishonest, invalidating, or disrespectful.

Press unpacks the idea in his book on patient satisfaction, written more than twenty years later:

> *Patients who are more satisfied are less likely to sue—period. All studies of malpractice claims show the same result. Communication is the key to the vast majority of suits. Anger, not injury, is the trigger for most claims.*[5]

Malcontent and malpractice

Press didn't know it then, but at the time there was another person coming to the same conclusion. Gerald Hickson, MD, a young pediatrician,

[5] Irwin Press, *Patient Satisfaction: Understanding and Managing the Experience of Care*, 2nd ed. (Chicago, IL: Health Administration Press, 2005).

was looking at the link between patient satisfaction and malpractice lawsuits in Tennessee. At about the same time Press was in Florida, Hickson earned a grant to study the reasons why patients sue their doctors.

Dr. Hickson graciously discussed the project with me. He said that the idea came to him after a discussion with an economist (Frank Sloan) who was interested in whether malpractice suits serve as a type of fringe health insurance for uninsured patients suffering from catastrophic illness or injury. He sought out families whose children had died or become permanently disabled in order to better understand why they sued their doctor.

Hickson, who is genuinely empathic and affable, with a slight southern drawl, recalled the main findings:

> *Families had a lack of trust in their physician. They perceived that the physicians did not care, and poorly understood their interactions. Many also felt they did not have access to information or their physician. Coupled with a poor outcome, families were more likely to sue.*

This sounds a lot like what was going on at Modern Memorial, as described by Press. Press and Hickson were both making similar observations at the same time, but Hickson, unlike Press, was an MD, which made him an insider. His findings would go on to be published in the medical literature rather than taught in college courses on anthropology.

Hickson remained in Tennessee where he helped formally implement changes to prevent the poor communication he saw with families who had lost a child. He did this after publishing the first solid link between malpractice and patient dissatisfaction. That evidence, unpublished at the time, was not yet available to Press, but it would become well known to hospital risk managers.

Risk managers become the catalyst for change

Press was still developing his ideas: that patients and physicians had different cultures, that this led to poor communication, and that failure to communicate increased malpractice risk. His feedback was ignored by the Modern Memorial physicians. If doctors wouldn't listen, then Press decided he would pursue hospital risk managers. They held a position of authority over the doctors and would be motivated by the increased risk of malpractice.

But like clinical medicine, Press knew little about hospital risk management. He wrote to the organizer of the brand-new American Society for Healthcare Risk Management. Their meeting was to feature a top malpractice lawyer who would speak on reasons why patients sue. It sounded perfect, but Press couldn't afford the fee to attend.

So he called the organization and explained, "I'm a professor at Notre Dame. I want to learn about risk management." So they gave him a 50 percent discount.

The day before the conference, Press realized he could, perhaps, offer something himself.

> *I wrote up a one-page summary of the relevance of cultural anthropology for hospital risk management. Just a one-page thing, maybe to hand out to people.*

Then he realized, as a consultant, he needed business cards. "I ran to a printer that I knew, and he said, 'I got a little machine over here; I can give you a dozen business cards right now.'"

The business cards read *Irwin Press, Anthropology Consultant.*

He left for Orlando the next morning. After a delayed flight, he rushed to his hotel and checked into his room, eager to change and get to the conference. He only had twenty minutes to spare.

"I'm in my hotel room; I'm late," Press says. As he's changing into his suit, the phone rings. It's the director of the society.

"She said, 'Our keynoter is fogged in Dallas, you're the only one who is different, would you mind addressing our group at noon?'

"So twenty minutes later, I'm addressing five hundred risk managers from all over the United States."

As a professor, Press wasn't a stranger to talking to large groups of people. He'd regularly taught classes of two hundred to three hundred students. But he wasn't used to the reception he got.

I was so different from anything they heard before, they loved it. The risk management newsletter that came out a month or two later referred to me as the dazzling star of the conference. As soon as the thing was over, all 12 of my business cards went out with the group. I got three invitations to speak at State Risk Management Society. A couple of weeks later I get a call from the Director of the Society: would I be the keynoter next year?

Overnight, Press became a key figure at conferences for hospital administrators and risk managers across America. Eager to find solutions to the worsening malpractice crisis of the early 1980s, they were captivated by Press. His message, and the new research linking malpractice and malcontent, sparked a movement toward using patient feedback to curb malpractice claims. Press approached Rod Gainey, his university colleague, when the time came to measure patient perception of care objectively.

As he recalls the growth of their company, he cannot remember a single difficulty. "We hired people to scale it up. Luckily hospitals were slow to sign up. We were hand pasting the charts together. It was a huge success. It was an idea whose time had come."

Today, Press continues to watch as the medical community reacts to policies that require a minimum level of satisfaction for full payment. It is a long way from being told that lacking an MD behind his name meant he couldn't understand the relationship between physician and patient.

In retrospect, it may seem unlikely that an anthropologist who started quietly observing patients and witch doctors would change the American medical system. I ask him about this while we conclude our time together. He shrugs and pushes up his glasses, unassuming and professorial. Press thinks little of this idea. He is, after all, just an anthropologist.

CHAPTER 5

BASICS OF PATIENT SATISFACTION, THE PRESS MODEL

I rwin Press, outsider to medicine, clearly saw the disconnect between patients and physicians. He then spent the majority of his career learning about what made patients appreciate their ED encounter, and what did not. As an anthropologist, the majority of his initial observations were about the different cultures of patient and physician. As a professional surveyor, he saw the practical ways to improve patient experience.

My time with Press was spent mostly talking about his career, but he also wrote a book, *Patient Satisfaction,* and published a white paper (available free online), "Strategies for Improving Patient Satisfaction with the Emergency Department Experience."[6] Based on his experience, he provides strategies to help improve patient experience.

Explanatory models and the sick role

As stated before, the difference in cultures between patient and physician is largely the result of different explanatory models. Specifically, between most physicians' strictly science-based closed model and most patients' all-inclusive open model, which takes into account factors like diet, life events, religion, and stress.

---

6 https://www.researchgate.net/file.PostFileLoader.html?id=55bf3c4a5dbbbd54c58b4580& assetKey=AS%3A273824094851073%401442296159702, accessed July 15, 2016.

The average patient's medical system...is open. To most of us, sickness is never an impersonal, anonymous event.[7]

Tied to the way we experience illness is the concept of the sick role. Throughout history, societies have had a role for the sick as part of different cultures, and when stricken people move into this role, it varies. Some move into this role only briefly, perhaps even concealing their sickness, while others might find themselves identifying more permanently with their illness. When a provider invalidates their patients' explanatory model or their sick role, it can make it impossible to form meaningful connections.

Expectations inform experience

Another aspect of patient satisfaction is the concept of expectation and hope. As patients, we carry to the ED certain expectations of how we hope things will be. It's the same for nonmedical experiences. Perhaps we expect to enjoy a movie, or for the audience to watch it quietly. Most people have low expectations of a dental visit, but high hopes for a birthday dinner. Previous experiences and beliefs give patients baseline expectations for their ED encounter.

Understanding that there are expectations, and hoping to meet or exceed them, is a concept borrowed by Press to help patients feel satisfied with their care. In the patient-satisfaction industry, this is referred to as the expectation-disconfirmation model:

Positive performance expectations met = satisfaction
Positive expectations surpassed = higher satisfaction
Negative expectations met = dissatisfaction
Negative expectations surpassed = satisfaction to highest satisfaction[8]

7 Irwin Press, *Patient Satisfaction*, 46.

8 Irwin Press, "Strategies for Improving Patient Satisfaction with the Emergency Department Experience," ResearchGate (2005), accessed July 15, 2015, https://www.researchgate.net/file.PostFileLoader.html?id=55bf3c4a5dbbbd54c58b4580&assetKey=AS%3A273824094851073%401442296159702.
Note: Paper was also shared with the author by Irwin Press in draft form prior to independent publishing, and is now available to public through its distribution by ResearchGate with the permission of Irwin Press.

Some suggest eliciting expectations from the patient at the beginning of their visit. The goal, then, would be to customize the ED visit to meet or exceed these expectations. Unfortunately, most patients aren't consciously aware of expectations they bring to the ED. They are focused on their illness, and rightly so. Most may not be able to provide information with enough detail and relevancy to make this a practical approach. Nevertheless, it's helpful to understand the concept that patients come with expectations and that meeting or exceeding those expectations creates a positive patient experience. Failing to meet them, on the other hand, disappoints.

Walking in the patient's shoes

Everyone sees the world through their own eyes, and each patient has unique expectations. Often they are quite different from their provider's. Some are primarily focused on pain control, whereas others are more interested in what their symptoms mean. What is their diagnosis? Is it dangerous?

Recall the patient Joy from earlier in the book. Her concerns were primarily the cause of her chest pain and whether it was dangerous. Her provider, John, would have a better chance of conveying value for the visit if he could learn her specific concerns and address them with her. Recall also that Joy's decision to come to the ED was difficult. Many patients agonize for days about the decision to come to the ED. Validating this decision helps the patient to put their doubts to rest. Press describes common patient concerns in his book:

> *Issues Underlying Patient Satisfaction with ED Care*
> 1. *Do I need to go to the emergency room?*
> 2. *Will they appreciate how stressful and inconvenient this visit is for me?*
> 3. *How do I get there?*
> 4. *Where do I go once I get there? Who do I see? What will happen next?*
> 5. *I'm embarrassed and don't want my visit and condition broadcast. Will staff respect my privacy?*
> 6. *Will I feel confident and at ease with the staff member who asks about my symptoms?*

7. *Will I be seen by a doctor immediately?*
8. *I arrived before other patients. Why are they being seen before me?*
9. *Why is this whole thing taking so long?*
10. *Do they realize how scared and stressed I am?*[9]

Press reminds us that patients often hope to be cured from their ailments, or at least to know the name of the disease. They want to be treated with respect and privacy, they don't want their complaint broadcast to the rest of the ED. Some patients fear that their problems have resulted from self-neglect or addiction, and they are wary of judgment or scorn from the ED staff.

They come with many questions: *Will my caretakers be kind? What if I'm hungry or need to get to the bathroom? Can my family be with me while I wait? How long will the ED encounter take, and what will I get for the time I invest?*

Press described contrasting provider priorities, like the ones experienced by our provider John, who treated Joy earlier in the book.

[Provider] Challenges:
1. *Stressful environment.*
2. *Mismatched views.*
3. *Disconnect in perceived acuity.*
4. *Conflicting therapy opinions.*
5. *Too little time.*[10]

As a provider you are responsible for, among other things, considering what's different today for the patient and what caused them to seek care. Other provider concerns include how fast our ancillary testing is carried out, a major source of pain in the ED. Providers are also charged with taking care of, not just individuals, but the community as a whole. This means attention to antibiotic stewardship and ED efficiency to quickly treat patients in waiting. Plus, you also need to eat and use the bathroom

---

9 Ibid.
10 Ibid.

during your shift. All these priorities are realities for providers, but they are not on the radar of most of your patients.

Legitimize, respect, and inform

In Press's model, these differences, combined with our cultural clash, create the difficulty in forming a meaningful connection. The problem he saw was failure by physicians to acknowledge these differences. He also felt physicians did not, as a group, recognize patient concerns as top priorities. Being the first voice to call attention to the situation, he was largely concerned with raising awareness. Recall that he believed showing physicians the problem would solve it for them. Once they understood, things could be different. He also developed a series of strategies to help providers do what he called "managing patient perceptions," another way of saying convey value. The strategies outlined by Press can be grouped (although not by him) into three actions: legitimize, respect, and inform.

Legitimize for Press means to help the patient understand their right to occupy their sick role and to have an open model of illness. He calls on providers to validate the decision to seek care in the emergency department and not to invalidate patients' explanatory model. He also describes the importance of the social and economic inconvenience of an ED visit, and understanding that the decision to seek care is seldom taken lightly.

Respect involves humane treatment; treatment that protects privacy and respects the patient. For example, as patients enter their room, it becomes their domain. We knock, ask to enter, give privacy, and allow families to be present. Respect, for Press, also means nonjudgmental when it comes to illnesses from self-neglect, addiction, and poor healthcare maintenance. Press notes that non-English-speaking patients have, on average, lower ED satisfaction. To effectively communicate and show respect, formal phone interpreters are required.

To keep the patient **informed**, we have to remember that they may not be acquainted with our ED rituals. Press suggests that the process of orienting the patient should begin before the visit with a user-friendly website, intuitive parking, and clear signs directing patients to the ED.

Everyone who speaks with the patient—including nurses, physicians, lab technicians, and radiologists—must inform the patient about what will happen next and roughly how long it will be until it happens. This information resets the patient's clock. "I've been here an hour and a half already" becomes "ten minutes to go before the doctor arrives."[11]

Information reduces stress, so orienting patients to different parts of their ED encounter helps people relax. How long they will wait and why? Patients feel more in-control when they know what is going to happen and can therefore be free to attend to other aspects of their visit. Press also makes a point of avoiding unpleasant surprises. Warn patients, because unexpected stress can be devastating, especially when they're sick. It is made easier when we can plan to endure the pain in advance. Press reminds us to give information about pain control and treatment, and to address the patient's hope for a cure, even if what we can provide is only reassurance.

11 Ibid.

CHAPTER 6

A SYSTEMATIC LOST IN EMPATHIA

I enjoyed my time with Irwin Press, but there is something I didn't share with him. From my perspective, I am very much a part of the culture of physicians he clashed with while at Modern Memorial. My training was at a large urban county hospital with poor resources and little time to forge meaningful connections, much less overcome cultural and language barriers. It wasn't hard to understand how interpersonal nuances could be lost in the daily crisis management. I had been part of the problem.

On one hand, I feel that Press's observations at Modern Memorial shine light onto the problem of why providers and patients don't connect, particularly in the ED. On the other hand, I also see levels of unappreciated complexity.

Statistically, it's unlikely that the stereotype "physicians are cold and uncaring" is true. Yes, there are definite differences in culture and beliefs between provider and patient. And forgive me for switching back and forth from provider to physician; there may be differences between the two groups in culture and perspective, but in each class of medical school, PA school, or nursing school, most applicants cite "helping others" as their primary motivation for going into medicine. If there was ever a group of professionals that might be viewed as altruistic, here it was. Volunteering and sacrificing only to work long hours for increasingly little reimbursement requires altruistic motivation.

If modern medical clinicians are viewed as systematic and uncaring, then please allow me to assert my thesis here: it's not because of who they are. The picture is more complicated than that.

The fundamental attribution error

The fundamental attribution error is a heuristic, or cognitive bias, that heavily influences our perception. Heuristics are cognitive shortcuts. Recall that, having survived the stone age, our intellects passed the natural selection process by parsing large amounts of sensory data quickly and organizing it so that we can make practical decisions. These quick practical decisions, called heuristics (literally: rule of thumb), become automatic.

The fundamental attribution error, also called in-group bias, is our tendency to attribute behavior to people's disposition rather than their circumstances. We find ourselves saying, "that's something he would do," rather than, "that's what any reasonable person would do, given the situation."

It's important because we are much more lenient when it comes to our own motivations, citing the situation, rather than those outside our social circle. It's a remnant of our days in tribes, helping the cohesiveness of the tribe by giving those in the social circle the benefit of the doubt. But in our modern society, where most people we encounter are not in our "tribe," it's nothing more than a bias.

Tribal origins of heuristic biases

Back in the tribe, when a large object in the woods moved a certain way, our ancestors reacted. Our reaction is now hard-wired because it was an evolutionary advantage to mistake a rock for a big black bear, whereas mistaking a bear for a rock usually only happened once, depending on the temperament of the bear.[12] These genetically based brain circuits al-

---

12 Metaphor adapted from: Nassim Taleb, *AntiFragile, Things That Gain from Disorder* (New York: Random House, 2012).

lowed our ancestors to make decisions quickly. Better circuits led to better decisions, which led to survival and the ability to reproduce: survival of the fittest brain. Cogitate to procreate.

Likewise, in our social lives we developed heuristics to better recognize our tribe members and survive within the tribal unit. They helped back then, but now are outdated quirks of our ancient brains. These quirks are maladapted to our modern environments, which partially explains why some patients prefer a traditional folk healer to a modern physician. Folk-healer methods evolved to meet the nonmedical needs of tribal members over thousands of years. It also helps explain why as medicine becomes more modern, it doesn't help providers and patients connect better. On the contrary, it seems that the more mechanistic and technology dependent we are at the bedside, the more disconnected we become.

> **The twentieth century was the bankruptcy
> of the social utopia; the twenty-first will
> be that of the technological one.**
> **—NASSIM TALEB**

Before we discuss the specific ways heuristics affect emergency medicine, let's explore the concept of heuristics and how they can affect interpersonal interactions.

Cognitive and optical illusions

Cognitive biases are to the brain what optical illusions are to our visual system. We take a quick glance and our visual system sometimes takes a shortcut, neuron to neuron, through an older part of our brain. Sometimes this works out for the best, and we see more quickly. Other times we make a mistake; a perceptual mistake. The optical illusion looks different than it is.

The Fraser Spiral[13] contains circles not a spiral, but the reality is lost to our visual system until you trace it with your finger.

Cognitive biases have been the subject of more research in the last two decades. This research is led by a group of psychologists, called behavioral economists, studying the tradeoffs concerning why humans behave the way they do.

13 *Figure: Fraser spiral illusion. Originally published by British Psychologist Sir James Fraser (1863 – 1936) in 1908. Adapted file (Public Domain) reproduced from Wikipedia, The Free Encyclopedia, https://commons.wikimedia.org/w/index.php?title=File:Fraser_spiral.svg&oldid=136598293. created by user Mysid, August 10, 2007/CC-BY-SA-3.0 (Accessed September 1, 2016)*

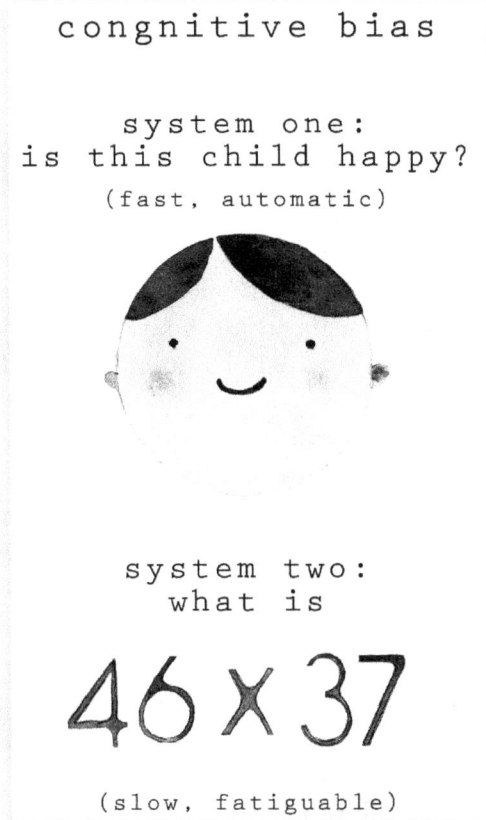

```
congnitive bias


system one:
is this child happy?
(fast, automatic)
```

```
system two:
what is
```

46 × 37

```
(slow, fatiguable)
```

At the root of these biases are two brain systems—not anatomical structures, but functional systems that include several variable anatomical locations. Cognitive Psychologist Daniel Kahneman calls them system one and system two.[14]

System one, the automatic system, is older, intuitive, and works effortlessly. It's the part of our cognitive machinery that guestimates. When we recognize genuine laughter, or see someone is about to lose their temper, this is the automatic system at work. It is also the system deceived by the visual trick in optical illusions.

14 Daniel Kahneman, *Thinking Fast and Slow* (New York: Macmillan, 2011).

System two, or the deliberate system, requires more effort. We have to intentionally engage and do the work. When we run our finger around the circles in the Fraser Spiral and see that they are circles, not spirals, that is our deliberate system. We also use it when we do long division or painfully multiply large numbers without guessing. In fact, any time you feel aversion to thinking about something, that is evidence you are using your deliberate system: practicing piano, doing taxes.

The aversion we feel to using the deliberate system can get us into trouble. This is where we begin to use heuristic shortcuts, system one, that bias our perception. They are fast, automatic, and don't cause mental fatigue.

For instance, it's much easier to conclude that, when someone loudly interrupts a meeting with false information, they simply aren't very smart; in other words, our conclusion is an oversimplification.

We are annoyed. But it could be, just as easily, that they are smart but making a mistake. Or that we are mistaken, and THEY are right.

To consider their situation, caffeine level, or the possibility that they were given bad information, is difficult because those are all harder questions to answer. It's not as easy to hold all those possibilities in our mind. It is much easier just to think: *that loudmouth is not so sharp.*

We answer the easier question as a shortcut and blame the person instead of their situation because of a heuristic, the fundamental-attribution error. And most times, we don't even realize what happened.

The cost of putting on a white coat

The question of what is at the root of the behavior of some physicians and providers is unclear. We are not all uncaring, but it's also not just biased thinking. There's more to it.

For instance, there is an undeniable effect of medical training on a person's disposition. Decety et al. examined brain fMRI scans of physicians versus nonmedical matched control subjects.[15][16] Subjects viewed

---

15 J. Decety, C.–Y. Yang, and Y. Cheng, "Physicians Down-Regulate Their Pain Empathy Response: An Event-Related Brain Potential Study," *NeuroImage* 50 (2010): 1676–82.

16 Y. Cheng, C.-P. Lin, H.-L. Liu, et al. "Expertise Modulates the Perception of Pain in Others," *Current Biology* 17 (2007): 1708–13.

videos of needles being slowly and painfully pushed into the finger-tips of strangers. Before training, students had average levels of fMRI-visualized activity in parts of the brain called the empathy circuit. This circuit is used when imagining what others might be feeling, including a section called the mirror neurons that is involved in imagining the physical pain of others. After medical training, the empathy circuit lit up less on fMRI when watching the same videos of needles piercing human fingers. Subjects still felt the pain of others, but the volume was turned way down.

Other studies have shown measures of empathy decline during medical training.[17,18] After training, the areas of these circuits had measurably less activity. This begs the question: What exactly are we trained to do?

For physicians and other providers in the United States, the situation has undergone radical changes, with more technology, in the past fifty years. Working as a provider today requires a command of computing, pharmacology, with a background in chemistry and math. We are now like engineers. Could it be that, as the demands of medicine became more technical over the last fifty years, recruiting has selected a more systematic healer?

The systematic-empathic spectrum

Simon Baron-Cohen, a British neuroscientist and cousin of the famous comedian Sasha Baron-Cohen, of Borat fame, studies the spectrum of empathic and systematic tendencies. In his book *The Science of Evil*, he describes variations in activity of individuals' empathy circuits. Some people have more active circuits than others when measured on an fMRI.

As a scientist, he's spent a fair amount of time investigating those who completely lack empathy. These include people with certain personality disorders and those suffering from psychopathy, who have no empathy. These subjects lack activity in the circuits of the brain that create an

17 M. Hojat, M. J. Vergare, K. Maxwell, et al. "The Devil Is in the Third Year: A Longitudinal Study of Erosion of Empathy in Medical School," *Acad Med* 84 (2009): 1182–91.

18 M. Neumann, F. Edelhäuser, D. Tauschel, et al. "Empathy Decline and Its Reasons: A Systematic Review of Studies with Medical Students and Residents," *Acad Med* 86 (2011): 996–1009.

emotional theory of the mind. Recall that theory of the mind means thinking about what others might be thinking. An emotional theory of the mind is the same, but just for emotional thoughts. For example, when you understand that a friend will be sad if you walk away upset, or that a person is angry because they were attacked, it's because your empathy circuit has constructed a mirror image of the other person's presumed emotional state of mind.

What Baron-Cohen has found is that everyone is different, ranging from the quirky to the pathological. Some people can easily imagine the world from eyes of others. Some cannot.

In some cases, a lack of empathy is balanced by an increased aptitude for understanding systems. For example, the autistic mathematical savant, or nonverbal child who draws intricate pictures.

This doesn't just apply to extreme examples. The spectrum also includes people who are just outside of the normal part of the bell curve. We see examples of this in everyday life: computer programmers with poor eye contact and social awkwardness. Or electrical engineers who might struggle as counselors, more systematic than empathic. It's like comparing machine efficiency to effortless sensing of emotions.

We all find ourselves somewhere on this spectrum. It's as though some of us come from a mythical land called Systemathia, where all the citizens are all systematically inclined. They can troubleshoot problems with their computers and assemble model airplanes without the directions. No one has trouble learning new software or hooking their new camera up to their new projector.

Over the mountains, in the bordering country of Empathia, live others who often need help with technical tasks but have no trouble communicating. It's not just what they say, either, but how they read each other's emotions. Sensing nonverbal cues, the people of Empathia don't interrupt each other. They know when the other person is waiting to speak, or doesn't understand. When you talk to someone from Empathia, you feel heard, and it feels good. Just don't ask them to help you defrag your hard drive.

As medicine has become more technical, systematic inclination puts applicants at an advantage. Information acquisition has become its own skill in modern premed programs. As we select for a more and more systematically oriented section of the population, we create medical professionals who become lost in Empathia.

Those medical providers of today who are indeed systematic may struggle at times to easily create an emotional theory of the mind. Not that we can't imagine what others might feel, but that there's a decreased aptitude in the effortless reading of nonverbal cues that help navigate the interpersonal dance with patients. Not having the same level of innate or learned ability, we are like robots with broken motion sensors, not knowing exactly when to stop. We are like emotional bumper cars.

Who we are and where we are: disposition and situation

Once aware of the fundamental attribution error, one wonders how much of provider and patient behavior is really due to disposition at all. In fact, psychology has struggled to demonstrate a basis for predicting people's behavior given testing on their disposition. Despite the popularity of personality tests, they have no value in predicting behavior.

The disposition/situation debate in psychology came to a close when, in 1968, American psychologist Walter Mischel mortally wounded the dispositionist theory in his book *Personality and Assessment*.[19] He cited research that showed an exceedingly low correlation (0.1–0.2) between actual behavior and predicted behavior based on personality testing of a person's friendliness, extroversion, tendency toward honesty, etc. If a person measured high for extroversion you could only predict they would act extroverted in a situation one time out of ten. After its publication, social psychology research began to focus on how circumstances affect behavior rather than the other way around. They abandoned the idea that we can predict what people will do if we know their disposition.

In contrast to the abysmal correlation found between disposition and behavior, research using experimental situations to influence behavior has been the foundation for social psychology over the last forty years. Consider the Milgram experiment, where subjects obeyed when led to believe they were delivering electric shocks to other subjects of increasing voltage. Situational bias affected subjects' behavior regardless of

19   Walter Mischel, *Personality and Assessment* (New York: Wiley, 1968).

43

their dispositions. Or the Zimbardo Stanford prison experiment, where subjects randomly assigned as guards became abusive. The situation was so powerful that the experiment had to be called off halfway through.

These experiments have demonstrated influencing people's behavior by creating experimental situations with built-in bias. Predicting behavior based on personality testing has been a flop, but because of our biases we continue to believe it works. In their book *The Person and the Situation*, Stanford psychologists Lee Ross and Richard Nisbett examine the last fifty years of research on the fundamental-attribution error. They describe the prevalence of public belief in personality testing and other measures of disposition. Ultimately, they conclude that behavior is likely a combination of situational factors and our choices in response to them, or an interaction of person and situation.

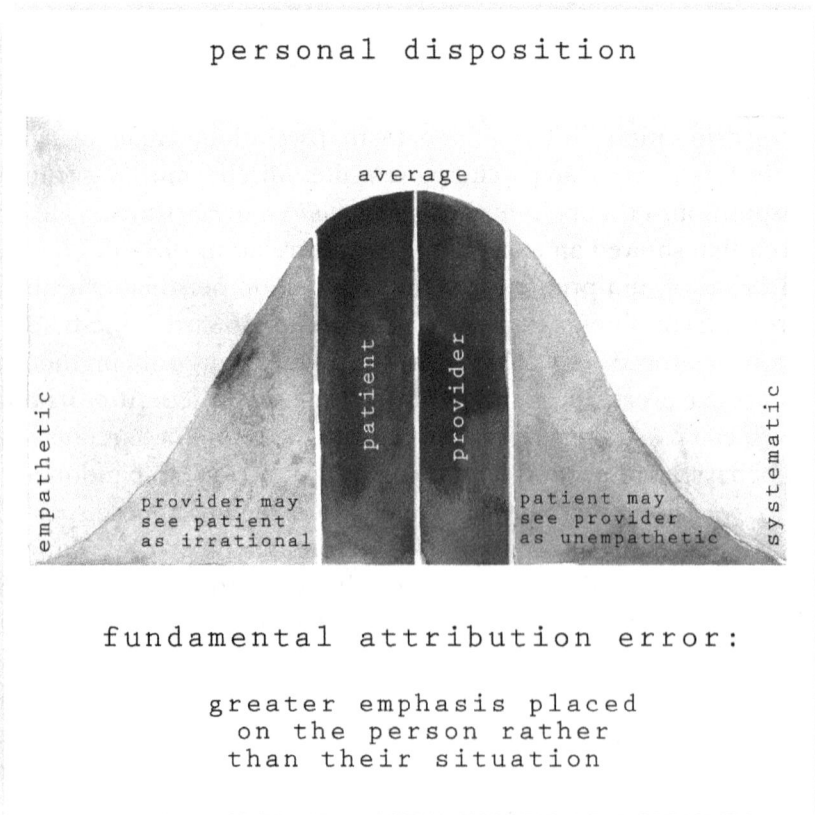

personal disposition

average

patient

provider

empathetic

systematic

provider may
see patient
as irrational

patient may
see provider
as unempathetic

fundamental attribution error:

greater emphasis placed
on the person rather
than their situation

The point is to ask: Does medical training make providers less empathetic toward the physical pain of others? Probably. Does the increasing technological demand of medicine lead to recruitment of more systematic people who are less adept at interpersonal subtleties? Maybe. How do people behave when we know their disposition? Psychological research says we have no idea.

What it does tell us is that our brains are better adapted to small tribes than big, modern social networks, and that we feel we know more about people based on what we see them do than we should. In this we are overconfident. Patients, who view providers carrying out our technical tasks, may view them as more systematic and uncaring than they actually are. And since no one is immune to the fundamental attribution error, providers may view patients as more emotional and less focused on the science when they refuse our closed model of illness.

What is the situational effect of taking care of other people? How does that effect interact with our systematics nature? Does the pressure to perform highly technical medicine while maintaining high productivity make us less helpful and personable?

How to blind Good Samaritans
The Good Samaritan Study was designed to evaluate "helping behavior" in the aftermath of the murder of Kitty Genovese which, in 1964, took place with multiple witnesses and allegedly little bystander intervention or calls to police.

Psychologists Dan Batson and John Darley were interested in the effect of the situation on behavior. Would you help someone in trouble, depending on the circumstances? They found that simply telling a subject that they were late, and needed to hurry, significantly reduced helping behavior. To date, it is the psychological study most relevant to provider behavior in the emergency department.

While I was researching this book, I had the opportunity to talk with Dan Batson about the Good Samaritan Study. Batson, kind and soft spoken, is an authority on the research of altruism and helping behavior. At the time of the experiment, he was finishing a degree in seminary, although he never entered the ministry:

Perhaps I'm an agnostic atheist… The God I believed in would be quite uninterested in what I believed, only in what I did.

Batson's area of study became differences between what people believed and what, ultimately, they did.

He took subjects from the seminary to see what they would do, presuming that they believed in the parable of the good Samaritan, who stopped to help someone in need who no one else would help on the road to Jericho.

Here is a shortened account from Gospel according to Luke, the only apostle who was also a physician:

> **A man was going down from Jerusalem to Jericho, when he was attacked by robbers. They stripped him of his clothes, beat him and went away, leaving him half dead. A priest happened to be going down the same road, and when he saw the man, he passed by on the other side. So too, a Levite, when he came to the place and saw him, passed by on the other side. But a Samaritan, as he traveled, came where the man was; and when he saw him, he took pity on him. He went to him and bandaged his wounds, pouring on oil and wine. Then he put the man on his own donkey, brought him to an inn and took care of him.**
> **LUKE 10:30–34**

The experiment took place at Princeton in winter. For subjects, Batson used forty male students from the seminary who were told they would prepare lectures either on the Good Samaritan (to prime for helping behavior in the style of a 1960s psychology experiment) or another "control" lecture. Then they were sent across campus with a map to another lecture hall to give their speech.

Here's the important part: half were told to hurry.

This, they hoped, would create another situational variable that might affect the choices of the subjects.

During their walk across campus, the subjects walked past an actor lying on the side of the road, like the victim on the road to Jericho in the story. The question was whether these seminary students, who had just prepared a talk on the Good Samaritan, would act as Good Samaritans themselves. Would they help a stranger who seemed sick in a cold alley on the Princeton campus? Or would they pass by on the other side?

Not all went as planned. At one point, a truck was blocking the alley they were using, obstructing the students' path. Later, it was so cold that the victim went inside to warm up and missed the students speeding by as they busily went over the lecture in their head while trying to find their way with the map.

In the end, Darley and Batson found that preparing a sermon about the Good Samaritan didn't affect behavior, but those who were made to hurry helped much less. Only one out of ten subjects in a hurry stopped to help. Control subjects not in a hurry helped much more often, 63 percent of the time. Regardless of who the subjects were or what they believed, when they were made to hurry, they became less inclined to help, significantly less.

Why would simply telling a subject they were running out of time cause them to miss the victim nine times in ten? Initial theories involved stress on the subjects' attention span or limiting the size of their cognitive map. Perhaps the added stress and surprise of being made to hurry caused them not to recognize that the victim needed help? Maybe being in a hurry made them less likely to see the victim altogether, or maybe just less inclined to help.

Helping ourselves to see clearly

I believe that the structure of the ED visit creates the same effect as Batson's Good Samaritan experiment. We become less helpful, and less attuned to the nonverbal communication of others, handicapping our interactions.

Knowing how situations affect behavior, how would we modify the ED "situation" to positively affect interpersonal interaction and the patient's experience of care? It's fast paced, and we are made to hurry. We are made to focus on the primary complaint and to consider other aspects of the patient less important. And we treat people who are, sometimes, having the worst day of their lives. But we do it all day, every day, and it becomes routine. While the Press model of ED care serves as an excellent foundation, we should go one step further. What if we could change the situation, the structure of the ED encounter to work with our heuristic nature, rather than clash against it?

CHAPTER 7

THE HEURISTIC MODEL OF CARE

In chapter 2, we saw that expectations for an ideal ED visit differ in the minds of most providers and patients. Each has different priorities and perspectives. Press might argue that these differences are cultural, but there is another layer of complexity. Our heuristic biases also affect our perception.

We are fooled by the ancient evolved machinery of our minds, preventing provider and patient from connecting. Providers mean well and are perhaps even altruistic, but the odds are stacked against them.

Press felt that adopting a customer-service approach to patient care would help make it more patient centered. But many providers find that, even after adopting this approach, patients often miss seeing the value in their care.

So how do we build the situation of the ED encounter to convey value so it isn't missed?

Fixing the structure of the ED encounter

Can we possibly be expected to fit all these details into an already complicated ED encounter? Providers barely have enough time to complete the review of systems and relevant exam, let alone address a whole host of other concerns. So how is it possible to cram all this in while moving at a responsible pace?

The answer is, quite simply, that there isn't enough time.

Don't stop reading.

The current ED encounter doesn't give you enough time with each patient to address all their concerns and make the perfect visit for everyone. Also, different patients want different things from their ED encounter; some want only a quick businesslike interaction, while other patients need counseling and support.

How would you design an ED encounter to help providers meaningfully connect with patients in a time-efficient way? You could start by taking out things that won't help. Luckily, much of what Press recommends are things we shouldn't do: judging, invalidating, criticizing. Each negative behavior you leave out means less wasted time.

Then, to optimize the time left over, make the most of moments that carry the most weight. Leverage fulcrumatic moments, and do it the same way each time using a checklist to build your habits.

So which moments are most important? Our heuristic bias makes some moments more important for recognizing value than others. Here are a few heuristic concepts that apply to the ED encounter:

The halo effect

When we first enter a patient's room, we make our first impression. How we look, our eye contact, and our introduction can provide lasting impressions that color the entire encounter.

Positive impressions help us connect with our patients because of our tendency to accept those we like into our own social groups or tribes, at least temporarily.

This is called the halo effect, and it's responsible for the added weight given to the patient's first impression of us. Ancient evolved structures in our brains help us quickly create an impression of another person through our initial eye contact. We sync like computers, but faster, and without cords. This first moment can be either really good for the interaction, or really bad.

Competency bias

After the initial contact, our patients begin to judge our competency. This is difficult for them because they are, presumably, not medical experts. But competency judging is not a new problem. Humans have had to judge the ability and intentions of others for our entire existence, and we have evolved a system to do it.

To make it easier, our minds take a shortcut called the substitution heuristic. Here's how it works. When it comes to answering complex questions, we often substitute an easier question for the more complicated one. For patients, often it's substituting a provider's ability to communicate for his or her medical expertise. This doesn't just happen in medicine. We all do it. Here is an example.

Once before a flight out of Denver in stormy weather I heard our pilot introduced himself over the intercom. He talked about the severe weather but also reassured us that he was a former Alaskan Bush pilot, accustomed to flying in bad weather. On top of that he had twenty-five additional years' experience flying commercial planes. He explained our flight would have heavy turbulence, but after his introduction we felt we were in expert hands. Before we took off, he was removed from the plane by security. He was intoxicated.

Why did we feel reassured? The pilot had excellent public speaking skills and a very refined speech to reassure his passengers. But how much crossover is there between public speaking skills and aviation? The answer is: none whatsoever. But that's how we've evolved to judge competency. We substitute attributes we can easily judge in place of those outside our expertise.

Patients may not know a provider's credentials or his or her level of experience. They substitute other aspects of the providers' behavior to judge whether they seem skilled or not. How do they listen? Do they convey clinical concern? Do they look professional and competent? Do they interact with the nursing staff in a respectful way? Show you're a competent communicator, and patients will want you to be their provider.

The asymmetry of negativity

Paul Rozin, world expert on disgust, might have you think of the ED visit as a bowl of cherries. He uses the metaphor of a bowl of cherries as a thought experiment to show the asymmetry of negative experiences.

Asymmetry, when positive and negative reactions are unequal, is a core example of heuristic bias. Our ancient minds evolved to survive, preferring to avoid rather than approach and flee conflict rather than risk loss.

This is called loss aversion, our tendency to avoid risk of loss over a chance at gaining something, even when they are equal.

Loss aversion can be mathematically measured in experiments. In general, losses tend to be twice as powerful, psychologically, as equivalent gains. They are asymmetric.

Rozin points out that a bowl full of succulent cherries is spoiled by a single cockroach, but a bowl of cockroaches does not gain appeal from adding a delicious sweet juicy cherry.

Another psychologist, John Gottman, claimed that in stable relationships, five positive interactions were required to balance a single negative one. He is famous in psychology for being able to predict if couples would divorce with 94 percent accuracy.

Negativity is more powerful than its counterpart.

Emotional concretization revisited

When we are sick, our brains often tell us that we will never get better. This doesn't always happen, but it can add to the pain and discomfort we already feel. Our hope that things will change for the better is sometimes overshadowed by an emotional inertia called concretization.

When you show genuine interest in patients' lives and who they are, you remind them that life goes on outside.

This is a little metaphysical, but they are stuck; you aren't, and you transfer your emotional inertia to them by showing them they are not alone. You help them become emotionally unstuck and provide hope that they will get better. It will help ease their suffering because they will know they are not alone.

The peak-end rule

The end of our visit also has added weight for coloring our perceptions. The peak-end rule is our tendency to more vividly recall the most intense moment and the final moment of any given experience. Those parts of the experience carry more weight in our memory.

This is because our minds are wired to remember the highlights and the end of experiences with more clarity and impact. Humans do not average their experiences equally when recalling an event. Rather they are asymmetrically influenced by key parts of the event.

As previously discussed, the ED is poorly designed for careful de-briefing of patients who we risk alienating at the end of their visit. We tend not to end the encounter very well.

Posterior plasticity

Human memory has a significant amount of plasticity. Postdischarge contact with the patient also has the potential to overwrite our memories with counterfactual ones—counterfeit memories that fit our narrative more than what actually happened.

When a patient receives an erroneous bill or a discharge phone call, his or her impression of the encounter is changed by the newly con-nected experience.

For example, perhaps you go on a blind date and no one shows up. You laugh with your server, decide not to waste the evening, and order food. It's the best meal you've had in years. Right before someone asks you about the meal, you find out that your date came to the restaurant, saw *you*, and left. Ouch. Was it still the best meal of your life? Maybe? But when you pass the restaurant, from now on, you will remember it differently.

Even a patient-satisfaction survey affects the memory of our ED en-counter. By asking about the encounter and having patients reflect, they access parts of the experience they most easily remember. For many it's easier to remember negative things, because they are unusual and make a bigger impression.

Calling your patients to touch base after the encounter has the same power to affect their memory of the experience and smooth over any rough edges. Can you imagine being called by your ED providers the next day to make sure you were OK and getting well?

Systematic inclination, the problem and the solution

The complexity of the interaction with patients in the ED makes improving our interactions difficult. Each encounter is unique. The provider balances interpersonal finesse with finding the medical problem and fixing it in the allotted time. As the provider makes efforts to meet all the demands, the improvement becomes somewhat asymptotic. Like bowling a perfect game, we get close, but it's hard to get it right in each frame.

That's the problem, but it's also the solution.

In order to consistently hit all the points, a provider has to use a systematic tool for an empathic task: an interpersonal checklist. The encounter has become too complicated and patients who will ultimately need more intensive interpersonal attention cannot be identified beforehand. Many of them will not tell us we are failing them, either. Studies suggest that fewer than 10 percent will complain. An empathic person might see the nonverbal cues, but not the systematic person, and not with everything else we need to do.

The ED visit must be time efficient. We have to balance managing perception with finding and fixing the patient's problem. Our systematic nature may blind us to nonverbal cues that the patient will be unsatisfied after discharge. For this reason, we match these fulcrumatic moments with a checklist to hit every important point every time, systematically. This is using our Achilles's heel as our arrow.

PART 2: THE CHECKLIST

CHAPTER 8

BUILDING THE CHECKLIST

Why use checklists in medicine?

"Kate...something's wrong...he doesn't look right. Sir...sir... Kate, I don't feel a pulse."

"Start CPR," Kate, our provider from earlier in the book, said as she was treating a patient with syncope when suddenly he became unresponsive.

"Wait, there's a beat...it's super slow."

The medics had just brought him in, and initially, he seemed fine. He was fine. Now he was crashing, his pulse too slow. Hypotensive, he passed out. He was in shock.

Kate froze for a moment. He had been talking to her, then looked ashen, staring. He looked dead. Before he crashed, she was about to go discuss the case with her attending. Now he was slipping through her fingers.

She needed to act, needed to get...to get...help—should she get help right now? He was bradycardic, maybe give him atropine first, right away, and then get help? What should she do first? She looked at the nurse...she was starting CPR, let her do that, and I'll...

Kate felt pulled in two directions. She was standing next to the patient's head with the nurse in front of her pushing on his chest, fast. There was equipment crowded all around them, she felt cramped and panicked. *He is going to die if I don't...*

Slammed in the middle of a crisis situation, everyone gets tunnel vision. Some people seem to handle it well. They hide their fear below layers of practice and experience. Everyone feels the pressure. Everyone freezes at some point.

Emergency medicine is unique because, at any time, things can go bad, and fast. A crisis like the one above would be less terrifying if it happened all the time, but it doesn't. It's rare, and that's what makes it hard.

If it happened more often, Kate would be ready. If she had recently treated a bradycardic patient, she would remember to first call for help, start CPR, give atropine, and then start transcutaneous pacing if atropine didn't help. She would have recently reviewed the common causes of bradycardia, and so she would know what to do next. But Kate hasn't had a case like this recently, unstable bradycardia is rare, and the therapy algorithm is complex. She is only human, and humans don't always perform complex tasks well. Enter the checklist.

Commercial pilots also have a complex job. When things go wrong, they go very wrong, very fast. The pressure is on because they may have over one-hundred people on their plane, and it's difficult to fix a high-stakes problem under pressure. The aviation industry knows this, and so they use volumes of checklists for different crisis situations. That way, when things go wrong, they can fix the problem even if they get tunnel vision and feel panicked. Pilots don't need to think about every step, and they won't risk missing an important one. Checklists act as a fulcrum to speed up the function of their cognitive system two, the deliberate system. When adrenaline dumps into their bodies, they, like everyone, have a tendency to default to system one, automatic. But a checklist puts system two on the fast track to fixing the problem.

———

"Behind you," Kate said as she slid behind the nurse. The crash cart was there and above it, on the wall, were the crisis checklists. She quickly traced one with her finger, scanning it. She was now the one engaging her deliberate system, like someone tracing the Fraser spiral optical illusion and seeing the circles for what they are...circles, not spirals—system two, not system one. Not fight or flight, but think.

The sign on the wall read:

Unstable Bradycardia
1. **Call for help and code cart**
2. **Turn oxygen to 100 percent**
3. **Give atropine**
4. **If ineffective, start transcutaneous pacing:**
   a. **Place the electrodes front and back**
   b. **Turn monitor/defibrillator to PACER mode**
   c. **Set PACER RATE (ppm) to 80/minute**
   d. **Start at 60 mA of PACER OUTPUT and increase until pacer spikes aligned with QRS**
   e. **Set final energy to 10 mA above initial capture level**
   f. **Confirm effective capture with palpable femoral pulse (carotid pulse unreliable)**

Kate turns and calls sharply for help. "Code Blue, room nine." She will need multiple people in the room with all that needs to be done.

She breaks open the crash cart and looks for the…there it is, atropine.

"I'll take that, thanks," she says as a second nurse steps in, her attending physician behind her.

"One mg of atropine injection."

The atropine doesn't work. Kate is looking at the checklist with her attending.

At the same time, Kate and her attending both say, "Pacer pads on."

They look at each other, and both turn to look at the patient. The nurses slap on the pads. Front. Back. They look back at Kate.

Kate then starts pacing the patient, who stabilizes and is saved. He was in acute renal failure, with a sky-high potassium of 8.1. A week later, after rounds of dialysis, he walks out of the hospital.

———

Getting things right every time
The checklist is your solution to the problem of complexity in modern medicine. To avoid missing a key step, medical teams now put those

steps into a list, made in advance with a cool head, before disaster strikes.

It's not only in crisis that checklists are useful. They also help you remember important things that are uncommon, like the big five life-threatening causes of chest pain:

1. **Acute coronary syndrome**
2. **Pulmonary embolism**
3. **Cardiac tamponade**
4. **Aortic dissection**
5. **Tension pneumothorax**

By listing the big five for each patient with chest pain, you consider these no-miss diagnoses each time. Then, when someone presents with a rare and lethal cause of chest pain, the list helps you recognize it.

When something is important, you need to get it right every time. So, ask yourself this question: Is the patient experience of care important? If it is, you'll find a way to use a checklist. If it isn't, you won't.

Can a checklist be applied in the ED?

You will fail to hit all the points without a systematic approach. An ED encounter cannot be done with a cookbook, but there is a recipe. If something is left out, an individual patient may not notice, but key steps will be missed. The result is that over time you will fail to meet your patients' nonmedical needs. During complex tasks, it's impossible to hold everything in your working memory. You need a plan to meet these needs each time, with little variance.

Here is an important point. Using a checklist is *not* scripting, or repeating memorized phrases while trying to sound sincere. Instead, it's a way, with your busy pace, to make sure you don't leave any issue unaddressed. Remember, the seminary students in Batson's Good Samaritan study didn't ignore the person on the roadside because they were cynical or uncaring. It was because they were placed in a situation with built-in bias. You can use that insight in the ED to show respect, keep each patient informed, and build rapport, every time.

Bridge of trust revisited

Recall the concept of the bridge of trust. Specifically, to reliably reassure patients at the end of the encounter you must build rapport early. At the end you'll ask them to trust you. But without adequately building this metaphorical bridge, all they'll see is an open gap with nothing to stand on.

Research on cognitive biases tells us that certain moments of the encounter carry more weight for building rapport. For example, the initial moment of your exchange is key. Once this impression has taken place, it has inertia. We call this inertia the halo effect. Whether patient perceptions are positive or negative, those initial perceptions will color the rest of the experience.

Remember also that patients who lack medical expertise tend to judge medical competency by the substitution heuristic. Specifically, they tend to substitute a provider's communication skills for medical expertise. This tendency is called competency bias. If you miss the opportunity to demonstrate competency early in the encounter, your bridge of trust will lack a firm foundation.

A third heuristic, the peak-end rule, tells us that two parts of the encounter profoundly affect the entire experience: the most intense part of the visit and its conclusion. After you take time to demonstrate competency –by exhibiting your superior communication skills– then you can begin to treat your patient. Hopefully, he or she will feel better. Symptoms will improve, and pain will lessen. If not, the patient may doubt your plan. If they feel worse, it may be hard for them to believe that you're making them well. The end of the encounter will also carry significant weight. Even if they feel better, it takes skill to close the encounter well, as we will see.

Our checklist must address these moments, and it should also have a step dedicated to expertly finishing the encounter.

Lack of time

Another consideration as we build our checklist is how little time we have with each patient. The ED is busy. Time is limited. Adding extra steps to fill in the gaps in patient experience is not always practical. Providers need to choose the right moments to focus on, strategically.

For example, spending time explaining why the ED is busy will prove less impactful than skillfully introducing yourself or thoroughly going over results at the end of a visit. Frequent contact has also been shown to shorten patient estimates of the length of their visit, while explaining how delays are the nurses' fault does not. That's a mistake. Another mistake is rushing patients with nonurgent complaints because of a heuristic called acuity dissonance, which is based on a concept known as the vertical-horizontal framework.

The vertical-horizontal framework

Let's revisit Joy, the young patient with chest pain at the beginning of the book. Joy had an intuition that her chest pain might not be life threatening and as a result she had many other concerns such as cost, whether she should be seeking care, and how disruptive the visit would be to the rest of her life.

When patients become more ill these concerns seem less important to them. If Joy becomes suddenly short of breath, the severity of her illness is, unfortunately, sharply validated. She starts to decompensate and her nonmedical needs disappear, erased by the threat to her life.

The customer service needs of a patient are often higher in patients with lower acuity. This is because of a concept called acuity dissonance.

In 1956, at Stanford, Leon Festinger described a related concept he called *cognitive dissonance*. He conducted an experiment where subjects were made to do tasks designed to be extremely boring. After the tasks, some subjects were paid a normal fee for their time, some nothing, and others only a dollar. Then they asked each subject to rate how interesting the boring task had been. For most subjects, there was no surprise. The task was designed to be boring, and it was...super...boring. But when they underpaid people, giving them only a dollar, psychologists were surprised by their findings.

Subjects who received only one dollar rated the task as significantly less boring, a seeming contradiction. Festinger hypothesized that this was because of the tension between the idea of having wasted their time on a boring task and the conflicting idea of not being well paid.

If the task is unthinkably boring, getting only a dollar seemed like a cruel joke, and subjects eased their inner conflict, which he called cognitive dissonance, by rating the task less boring in retrospect.

Here is where cognitive dissonance relates to lower-acuity patients having relatively more pressing nonmedical needs. Patients, just like everyone else, experience cognitive dissonance. Sometimes they feel it in the ED when two ideas conflict about their acuity. The decision to seek care is not an easy one. People hesitate to make themselves a burden to the ED, or to their family members who came with them. When they misjudge their emergency, they experience cognitive dissonance about their acuity, or more specifically, *acuity dissonance.*

They might believe on a subconscious level: I'm a reasonably tough person, but I just came in to waste time and money on an ED visit for a minor complaint. These two beliefs contradict.

The contradiction creates tension, just like it does in other areas of our lives. For example, the contradiction that I'm honest, and yet I cheated on my taxes creates a feeling of guilt. I'm punctual, and so when I'm late, it creates tension, and we create an excuse in order to feel we are late for a good reason. We are late because of traffic, not because we are habitually tardy. Sometimes we are aware of this tension, sometimes not.

In acuity dissonance, if patients are made to feel they have sought care inappropriately, then in order to resolve this dissonance they may subconsciously feel the need to receive a greater value in the ED in order to get their money's worth (or time's worth). Validating patients' reasons for seeking care helps them feel better about their decision. It diffuses the tension. Invalidating their decision draws wrath. It destroys rapport.

The effect of complex emotions is higher in less acute, or vertical patients. Sick, horizontal patients do not struggle with their decision to seek care. Large investments in customer service for sicker patients are not always appropriate, but they desperately need to be kept informed and treated in a patient-centered way. Most of our energy needs to be focused on their medical stabilization, and patients understand that.

The point of the vertical-horizontal framework is that when your patients have low acuity, they still have nonmedical needs, even though their medical needs may be easy to meet. Their nonmedical needs are legitimate, so rushing them through their encounter is a disservice. Inexperienced providers make the mistake of ignoring nonmedical needs at their peril.

When you decide to make your patient's perspective a priority and do things in a systematic way, you won't always see improvement, but it will be there. Your perspective is too intimate to see the big picture. Like looking at our face in the mirror every day, you won't notice small differences. But change is the only constant. Each day your practice habits evolve, one direction or the other. You get to choose which way. As you change habits, the work will seem harder at first. You will feel the emotional labor of intentional practice. Then, after time, it will get easier. Then it becomes automatic.

CHAPTER 9

THE CHECKLIST

I f your only priority was to create an ED encounter that conveyed the maximum value, and you had no restraints, you would radically change the encounter. It would start with a powerful introduction to show your patients and their family that this was the highest quality facility, with a provider who holds impeccable credentials. Do I hear Bach? A single private room, diplomas on the wall, spotless, warm, and cozy… there is no way that would ever happen in a busy ED.

Next, you would have your patients tell their story while carefully listening as a scribe diagrams their symptoms on a white board behind you, organizing them carefully. You would create a plan with them, and orient them to the details of their visit. While they waited, you might address the needs of their family: "Coffee or tea? Perhaps a biscuit?"

Then you would enter with your team: the lab technician, the radiologist, and your attending physician. Each member would take turns presenting the data. You would summarize the findings and their implications for patients and the families, using visual aids displayed on a giant flat-screen TV. After carefully answering all their questions, you would give your patients a bound report of the findings and their customized plan. It would, of course, also be sent via FedEx to their primary doctor, who had participated in the encounter via teleconference, but kept mercifully quiet.

There is just no way, right?

So how do we strike a balance between taking care of all our patients and meeting the medical and nonmedical needs of each individual in a reasonable way? After my time with Press, Hickson, and other gracious people who helped with this book, I came to the conclusion that a checklist must be short, specific, and involve only the nonmedical needs that can be reasonably addressed in a fast-paced ED.

The Checklist: (each step addresses a nonmedical need)
1. Competency judging: create the best first impression possible
2. Let them tell their story: meet the patient's need to empty their working memory of all the HPI details
3. Take a social history with clinical curiosity
4. Orient the patient to their visit: satisfy the need for information
5. Finish Big

Step 1: Competency judging

Recall that competency judging is subject to a heuristic bias known as substitution. People watch what we do and use this information to decide if we do it well.

Positive perception begins with preparation. Most patients will expect their physicians to have done their homework on the case before entering the room. They expect their medical records to be reviewed and assume the information they gave to the triage and intake nurses has been conveyed to the provider.

Many of our patients wait a long time to see a provider, and you might be tempted to rush in to minimize their wait; but remember that this initial moment is important. As you enter the patient's room, you sync with your patient and either gain a degree of grace, known as the halo effect, or fail to do so, and spend the rest of the encounter playing catch up.

The halo effect heuristic requires that you take a moment to familiarize yourself with the patient's case, medical records, and nursing notes. Not only is this good medicine, but you can also get a heads up from the nurse if this promises to be a difficult interaction. You can go in prepared.

As you enter the room

Patients and providers, being human, judge a book by its cover, at least initially. Western culture dictates that competent physicians look a certain way. Studies on the subject suggest that scrubs and a white coat are equal to business attire in terms of looking professional, so the least we can get away with is scrubs.

Earlier, I alluded to syncing with a patient, like a computer and a smartphone. Our ancient minds connect with others just like the connections of Internet-protocol software, but instead of plugging-in, we use a wireless signal: our eyes.

Making solid eye contact and taking a moment to connect help our patients accept us into their tribe. First impressions have inertia, positive or negative, so it's best to make a human connection before you log in to the actual computer at the bedside.

Social proof

After entering and sitting down (sitting down is very important every time we go to the bedside), a formal introduction to everyone in the room helps establish authority and set the tone. Introduce yourself to family members to harness their social proof, our tendency to judge situations by the opinions of those around us. If your introduction to the patient's family is fumbled, the patient experience will suffer. The family's opinion of the provider is important to the patient.

Venerating your team

Say something positive about the other members of your team, such as the nurse and the tech in the room. Commonly referred to as "venerating," or "managing-up," this builds the patient's confidence in the cohesiveness of your tribe. Cohesive teams are quality teams. When patients see people working together in harmony, they feel at ease.

Checking two patient identifiers helps project patient safety as a priority, and explaining why you are drawing the curtain (for privacy) helps patients register your concern for their dignity.

Gaining admission to the tribe

We want the people we adopt into our informal tribes to be similar to us. In medicine, we risk alienating patients by using medical jargon and ambiguous language. It's also important to recognize that while the use of formal language keeps us out of trouble, we need to keep our explanations straightforward and easy to understand. Patients sometimes misunderstand our medical doublespeak. When they feel excluded by the jargon, it fails to keep us in their tribe. Press also pointed out in his book that it helps to avoid vague statements such as "what's good for the goose is good for the gander," as ambiguity often makes people feel uncomfortable.

Professional telephone interpreter services are now readily accessible. They should be used in all cases where there is a language barrier; don't use family members as interpreters for a multitude of reasons beyond the scope of this book.

Step 2: The patient's story

Chronologic recall

Taking a patient-centered history is another important moment, and how we do it matters. Information is stored chronologically in the human brain. When events happen, we sometimes know we will need to tell the story later, but not always. Some patients carry a notebook and write all their symptoms down, but most people can't easily recall all the details. When eliciting a history, it's easier for the patient to recall the events in chronological order as they happened, so let them tell it that way.

Listening to the whole story, told from start to finish, is a hard way to get the medical information we need as providers. While the sequence of events can sometimes suggest a diagnosis, we need specific details. It's tempting to interrupt. Studies show most of us interrupt in the first few minutes.

For your patients, the interruption is not only disruptive to their storytelling, but also interferes with their ability to empty their working memory. When patients are first brought to their room, they usually have full bladders and full working memories. They want to tell their story, start to finish, and they want to use the restroom.

Only after patients have relayed all the details they feel are relevant, and they feel the peace of completely unloading them, will they be able to hear what you have to say. People sometimes feel anxiety about leaving out subtle details that you might use to tie all their symptoms together, in a single syndrome. From a layman perspective, with an open model of illness, any detail could be important.

Open questions

Open questions help patients tell their story. Sometimes we need to draw attention to the fact that their working memory is nearly empty with a phrase like, "I hear you saying...is there anything else going on?" Avoid the yes/no checklist that often leads to pigeonholing a diagnosis. When patients digress into the psychosocial aspects of their illness, they often do so for a relatively short amount of time. Allowing them to get through these details uninterrupted preserves social capital. You never know when you may need to cash it in, so save it all.

Interruptions

While obtaining a patient's history in a busy ED, you might be busy, too. For you, interruptions are routine, but your patient may not understand what is happening outside his or her room. Briefly explaining the basic nature of the interruption, without violating confidentiality, helps your patients understand the situation. They can then refocus on relaying their history without becoming emotionally derailed. Communicate to them verbally and nonverbally that they are your priority: keep eye contact, use neutral body language, and don't check your watch, unless you're taking their pulse.

Step 3: Clinical curiosity during the social history

As part of taking the patient's history, providers take a social history, habits that may contribute to comorbid illness: tobacco, alcohol, and drug use. This moment between provider and patient is profoundly important. Most of us just gloss over it, and that is a huge missed opportunity in emergency medicine. When patients come to the ED it can be the worst day of their life. Their health and happiness are at risk, and their lives are disrupted. Often this feels, to our patients, like things are going wrong, and will never change.

Emotional concretization revisited

As stated previously, patients suffering negative emotions sometimes experience a feeling that their negative circumstances are set in stone. This response to illness is described by Jodi Halpern in her book *From Detached Concern to Empathy*. Halpern uses the word *concretization* for patients who lose their sense of self-efficacy.

> *In a concretized emotional state the person's view...in the world is distorted. Instead of developing a view based on openness to evidence, he fits the evidence to a view.*[20]

This top-down view casts a shadow over the ED experience. It is another heuristic, a trick on the brain where patients feel trapped. The medical model of detached concern, as discussed earlier, warns against emotional involvement with patients, but complete detachment is impossible. Contemporary cognitive theory suggests that emotions are irreversibly bound to other aspects of our cognition. On their worst day, your patients may depend on their provider to help them overcome emotional concretization—not minimizing or ignoring the emotional aspect of their suffering. Halpern calls this emotional support of patients "nonabandonment."

In order to reclaim control of their life, patients need you to help them remember that their future is not determined by their illness and that their world will be sufficiently responsive to their efforts. You are present with them in their suffering. As providers, you reinforce their

---

20 Jodi Hapern, *From Detached Concern to Empathy: Humanizing Medical Practice* (Oxford: Oxford Press, 2001).

self-efficacy. You show empathy through your own curiosity about their humanity.

The goal of the social history is not to blame patients for being self-destructive. Do you smoke? Do you drink? The goal is to learn about them: Who they are? And what they love? Then to remind them that no matter how devastating the day feels, it too will pass, and that we, their providers, will not abandon them.

Clinical curiosity is empathy

How does this look from a practical point of view? As providers, we need to meet patients where they are, emotionally. In the ED, you are not required to perform a full counseling session, but you can show genuine interest. This can be as simple as asking what they do for fun, and you can do it while you begin their exam.

Many patients, when asked this simple question, will have no answer at first. Their reticence is actually the heuristic bias of emotional concretization, convincing them, in their illness, that nothing they do is fun.

"Nothing," they often say, at first. But gently probe into their lives, and they open up. As disruptive as serious ED encounters can be, most visits are only moments in our patients' lives, nothing more. But it doesn't always feel that way to your patients. As their healer, you give your patients the strength to know the truth, that dawn will come, and the storm will pass.

Putting the ED visit in context

From the provider's point of view, most ED complaints seem to be low acuity. We get used to the day-to-day routine and forget about the perspective of our patients. They are not used to our routine.

Patients may not know if their complaint is time sensitive. It could mean life or death. They may have an idea that they will be all right, but in life nothing is promised. Their friends may have suffered illnesses, become disabled, or even died without warning. From their perspective, it's better to get checked out; better safe than sorry. Our familiarity with the ED routine does not comfort them.

On top of this, emotional concretization, the feeling that the current illness is here to stay, can make the situation seem worse. Uncertainty, fear, and concretization set the ED visit up to be a negative experience.

Some medical and nursing professionals make the mistake of trying to put the low acuity of patients' complaint in context for them. They tell their patients, in what they think is a reassuring way, that they will be just fine, things will get better, and maybe they would have gotten better even if they hadn't come in. This is hard to hear. Acuity dissonance creates tension in patients' mind. The belief that they would only seek care in an emergency conflicts with the fact that they sought care for a minor complaint. Telling patients that they shouldn't have come to the ED is usually a mistake.

Rather than putting their problem into context by telling them their problem is low acuity, consider using the social history to provide that context indirectly. Having a moment to connect about the more positive aspects of your patients' lives, like what they do for fun, their children, and their passions, helps them access less dark areas of their minds. It reminds them about the rest of their life and puts the ED visit in context without creating cognitive dissonance and frustration.

Do they love to read to their grandchildren? Let's get them back to it. The patient is a green-thumbed gardener with back strain? Time to get the patient on the road to recovery so that she or he can get back to the garden.

Connecting with patients about what makes them unique shows empathy through genuine curiosity. Choosing to be curious about other parts of the patient's life taps into a deep, tribal need to feel unique; and our patients are unique, but we need to recognize it. When we take a moment to learn about our patients, it helps them reinstate their self-efficacy, empowering them to get better. They will get better, but just saying it doesn't help. By conveying genuine interest, we show them.

Patient-centered medical decision making

After taking an expanded social history to connect with our patients, it's time to discuss our treatment plan; involving our patients in the process shows that we value their autonomy. Often providers are frustrated by patients' investment in their own open models of illness, making it difficult to come to an agreement about how best to scientifically approach diagnosis and treatment. This is complicated by the body's tendency to repair itself, making self-treatment seem effective.

Success of patients' explanatory models and self-treatment is heavily supported by the body's tendency to constantly restore itself, explained here by Irwin Press in his book *Patient Satisfaction*:

> *The reason self-treatment is so universal is that is typically works. The vast majority of sicknesses are self-limiting. No matter what you do for it, you eventually recover and give credit to the remedies you used at home.*[21]

Take a moment to discuss your plan with the patient and explain your concerns. A brief conversation about differences in what you both think the patient needs can help unearth patient expectations, if he or she has any. What is the patient concerned about? What, specifically, is the provider concerned about? Are your patients at risk for pulmonary embolism or pneumothorax? What testing will they need to address these concerns?

The white-elephant problem

William Bradshaw, PhD, a biologist studying, among other things, genetic adaptations to climate change in nature, sometimes cited a thought experiment in his teaching. He would begin with a bar-room joke:

"Do you know how to kill a purple elephant? Well, with a purple-elephant gun, of course. And so how do you kill a white elephant?"

To which many answer, "A white-elephant gun."

Nope.

"You take the white elephant and tie its trunk in a knot, and when it turns purple, use the purple-elephant gun. Everyone knows that."

In the ED, we are constantly making white elephants into problems we can address and customizing care. Patients are sometimes frustrated

---

21 Irwin Press, *Patient Satisfaction*, 46.

when their problem is not easily fixed in the ED. We can't be all things to all people. But what we provide *is* quite valuable: an expert judgment as to what may be causing the patient's symptoms, whether it is dangerous, and how best to access the medical system to get what the patient needs. Patients can miss this value, but having a discussion to develop what they need and what we can do to help them increases the chances they will see it.

Step 4: Orient the patient, satisfy the need for information

Most patients have no idea what to expect. Remember, what is routine to us is novel to them. They don't know what information you get from their physical exam or what you're looking for. Giving them information helps ease their stress. A brief synopsis of what you have planned for their visit gives THEM a sort of checklist, and it helps them relax. They will appreciate that you kept them informed. Wouldn't you?

Orient your patients to what will happen during their visit

"Let me tell you what will happen next. First Jack, the tech here, will draw your blood using an IV. There's a needle but he takes it out, and then it's just plastic, so you can bend your arm. We'll use that IV to give you medicine and fluids. While you wait, your blood will go to the lab where technicians will check your blood and cardiac levels. I'll review them with you later. Another person will take you into another part of the ED, where we will take two x-rays of your chest. It takes about fifteen minutes; then you'll be back here. Altogether it will take us about two hours to get done with two days' worth of tests. While you wait, I'll be going over your tests with the attending physician. It's important to me that you stay informed. Do you have any questions?"

Frequent check-ins

Most ED managers recommend that providers check on their patients every fifteen to thirty minutes during their visit, even if tests are not back. Again, studies have shown frequent checks may cause patients to feel that wait times are shorter than they actually are, and it shows our concern. It's easy to feel ignored in the frenetic ED:

I don't have all your results yet, but I wanted to check in. If I were in your shoes, I would want to know what's going on so I'll keep you in the loop.

Empathy, reciprocity, and accountability.

Step 5: Finish big, and help the patient remember the value of their ED visit

Ending well in the ED takes discipline. The ED is set up to see people quickly, and then find and intervene with life-threatening conditions. Everything in the ED is set up to optimize the front end of the experience. But when it comes to conveying value, the most powerful moment is at the end.

Ideally, your conclusion should involve an efficient summary of the whole encounter. You must sit down and review the initial reason your patients sought care. Then, take time to go over all the results with them, whether or not they were normal, to help them attend to the thoroughness and depth of their evaluation. Address any conversations with specialists or nurses, show them their x-rays and labs. Discuss the life-threatening diagnoses that you considered and ruled out. Time invested at the end is more powerful than during any other part of the visit.

Daniel Kahneman describes a heuristic called the peak-end rule, where people tend to recall the peak of an experience, and its end, better than the rest. In his book *Thinking Fast and Slow*, he describes an experience where patients underwent a colonoscopy and rated their discomfort during the procedure. Then, after the procedure, they were asked to rate the overall experience in terms of discomfort. Overall ratings tended to correlate with the end of the procedure or the peak. If the procedure was long and unpleasant but ended well, it was rated more positive. On the other hand, short, easy procedures with painful endings were rated more negatively.

Many of us have had the experience of an event recast by a poor ending. We are out on a summer evening enjoying dinner. We are seated promptly, our server is polite, and he brings us a brilliant wine that exceeds our expectations. Dinner is also a pleasant surprise, and we sit in the afterglow awaiting dessert. We wait, and we wait, but nothing happens. When we inquire, we find that our server actually left at the end of his shift and did not switch our service to anyone else. An unapologetic staff member drops the dessert into a box, and we rush home late to relieve the babysitter. Would we have a different story of the evening out if dessert had come the way it always has, promptly, with the check and refills of water glasses?

Reassurance

Much of what we do in the ED is to reassure patients that their symptoms, while valid and unpleasant, are not dangerous and largely self-resolving. Many patients feel a fair amount of anxiety about their symptoms and long, subconsciously, to be given the name of an illness or syndrome to explain why they don't feel well. By naming their illness, we have shown them their enemy. When we fail to do this, patients can feel very unsatisfied.

In this situation, it can help to acknowledge that our tests, while powerful for detecting life-threatening conditions, are not perfect. Patients have to not only listen to their body but must also realize that, although something is going on, and they aren't well, it's not dangerous, and for that we are grateful.

Patient teaching

The end of our encounter is also an excellent time to give patients information they might need to navigate their course back to becoming well again.

Teaching should be short and simple. Use basic concepts and vocabulary, but no jargon. Also respect their medical knowledge. You can take care of either situation by saying, "You may already know this, but…"

Patients usually only remember one thing from the end of the visit, so make it count. Avoid metaphors or any vague concepts. Try to end the encounter on an energetic high point. Show them you are grateful for having the chance to participate in their care.

Contact after the encounter

The final major hurdle for patient perception in the ED encounter is the plasticity of human memory. The posteriority complex is a heuristic that refers to our plastic memories' tendency to rewrite our experiences in retrospect. It can create counterfactual memories of events, depending on what happens afterword. Calling your patients at home can help remind them of the value of their visit, make sure they understand the plan, and confirm their intention to follow through with it.

Practical checklist in action

To give a concrete example of a systematic approach to meeting the patient's nonmedical needs, consider the following:

1. Establish competency: an intro with credentials to harness the halo effect is important.
2. Unpack: unburden your patients' working memory by letting them tell their story uninterrupted and chronologically, not because it's efficient, but because it's important.
3. Connect—use the social history to break emotional concretization.
4. Partner with your patients: develop a plan out loud and goals for the visit. Orient patients to their visit, and talk through exam, and tell them what to expect.
    Emergency medicine is a contact sport: contact your patients early and often while they wait for their results, but keep it brief.
5. Finish big: Harness the power of the peak-end heuristic.
    Plan for the future together: when appropriate, let your patients know they can call the ED to decrease anxiety.
    Afterword: Consider contact after the encounter to make sure things are going as planned for your patients.

By adapting the steps of the checklist to meet your own personal style you will make it even better. The purpose is to intentionally set aside time during the encounter to make patient centeredness a priority.

When we make time to connect, it helps create a therapeutic partnership. Creating positive perceptions highlights the work we put in while taking care of each patient.

PART 3: THE TRIBE

CHAPTER 10

OUR TRAGIC FLAW

*Education is an admirable thing. But it is well
to remember from time to time that nothing
that is worth knowing can be taught.*
—OSCAR WILDE

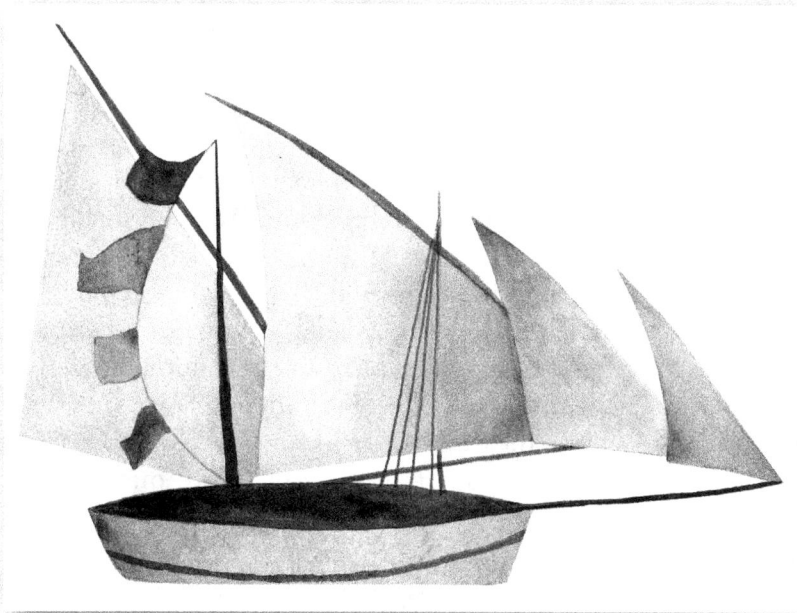

I like to sit by the fire with my little boys and tell them bedtime stories. Every story has a hero, and while I make one up each time, they already have one in mind. I can see it in their unblinking eyes. He's not a perfect hero, and he's not a bad person, but someone in between. He is complicated. The hero's life is in harmony and everything seems to be going well. That's not much of a story, so I make it interesting. The hero has a tragic flaw, something that will ultimately make their story a tragedy or an adventure. Whether it's a triumph or tragedy depends on whether the hero will learn about their flaw too late, or just on time. Will the hero's epiphany come before the final test? The boys will usually just settle for some kind of sword fight.

Medicine in America has been heavily influenced by American values of independence and self-reliance. Our heroes are men like Louis Pasteur, who took a risk and gave the rabies vaccine to a nine-year-old boy, saving his life against all odds. Emergency medicine is among the most independent specialties. We have become so independently skilled that most hospitals depend on ED physicians to carry out lifesaving procedures in the ICU and on pediatric floors. At times we are the heroes, but we also have a tragic flaw. It's our independence.

This final section of the book is about you, the provider, but it's also about your team. Although independence is a major cultural value in our modern medical culture, I think you will find, just like other areas of modern medicine, that something has been lost in becoming modern. There is a catch-22 where, in the modern world, technology enables us to be more independent while the complexity of modern medicine is too much for a single person to handle alone. We need our team, but that's not the way most of us were taught.

In American medical training, we are first heavily reliant on our teachers. Without their help and supervision, we are lost. Then, at some point in our training, we are encouraged to go it alone. Students take ownership of their learning and become independent. They become providers. Ownership is the key step to assume responsibility for their patients' care. To complete our training, and begin our practice, we must go it alone.

Our independence, the tool that helps us so well in learning medicine, sabotages us in our day-to-day work. During training, our ability to work alone helps get the job done. The information we learn builds the foundation for our skills. Later, as we enter the ED and join our new team, the complexity demands different work habits.

The truth is that even Louis Pasteur was not completely independent at the bedside. He had another person perform the actual injection for his rabies vaccine. Pasteur was a microbiologist, not formally trained or licensed as a physician. By using other members of his team, he could be assured that problems with the injection, like antisepsis, would not interfere with his primary goal of saving the child from fatal rabies.

The ship model

Imagine the hero Odysseus sailing his ship across the Aegean. He fights monsters and outsmarts the Cyclops, but aside from the heroics, he has basic practical needs for his voyage. The hull of the ship must withstand the stress of storms, his crew needs to work efficiently to operate and defend the vessel, and the sails have to be trimmed to catch the wind so he can escape danger.

Our ED strategy for conveying value is also like a ship. As Hickson and Press described, negative experiences can destroy all positive efforts during our encounter and make any improving the experience of care impossible. Using a checklist in our interpersonal interactions helps trim the sails of our boats, so we can sail smoothly through the stormy chaotic ED. But many of us have holes in our boat that can bring progress to a halt. These negative behaviors are deal breakers, and our own cognitive biases often prevent us from seeing them, at least in our own behavior.

Holes in our game can include lack of emotional control. Many providers spend very little time learning conflict resolution. We often avoid conflict, and when forced to navigate it, we fumble. Our systematic nature makes us less adept at forming an emotional theory of the mind in order to predict others' emotional states and how they will react. We don't know where to tread lightly. Being good at the systems of medicine may mean being bad at reading nonverbal cues of others. We don't see the signs and can be emotional bulls in the metaphorical china shop.

Other deal breakers include abusive behavior, verbal berating, condescension, and outbursts of anger at work. Patients use their substitution heuristic to judge our competency based on what they see, and poor interactions between providers and nurses speak volumes. Victim blaming is another gaping hole. Our brief time in the lives of others gives us limited insight into their situation, and judgment destroys rapport.

Sexual harassment, sarcasm, and cynicism are also deal breakers. Alcohol and drug dependence are deal breakers. Chronic tardiness, obstruction to change, and being a poor team player literally break the deal. They violate the unwritten agreement we have with other members of our team, just like gossip or character assassination. These are all holes in the ship that will sink it if given time. No amount of scripting or communication training will matter if there are holes like this in your game. They can destroy all your hard work.

CHAPTER 11

GERALD HICKSON AND MODERN MEDICAL PROFESSIONALISM

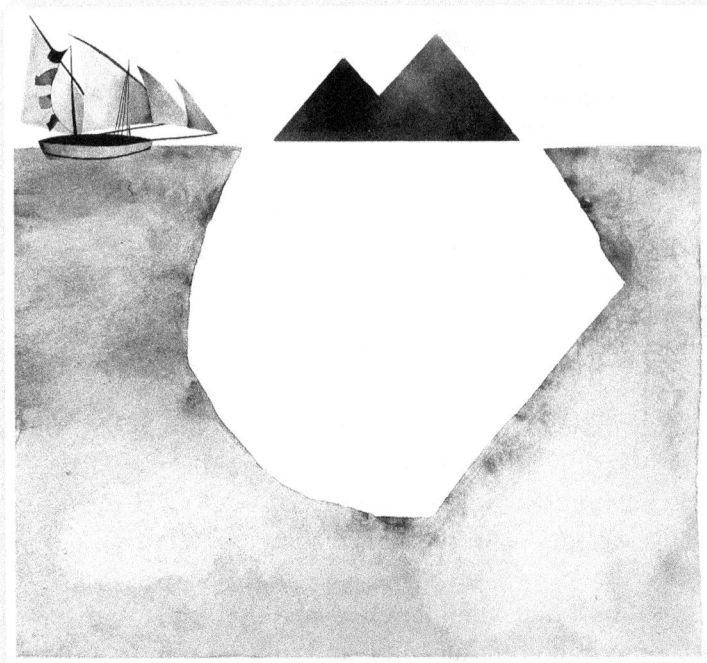

Holes in the boat

What happens when a community directly addresses disruptive behavior? How do things change when we refuse to tolerate the kind of habits we might call "holes in the boat" such as verbal abuse, lack of accountability, and refusal to practice in a patient-centered way? Gerald Hickson, the pediatrician who began his career studying why patients sue their doctors, created a program at Vanderbilt focused on giving patients a voice. He called it the Center for Patient and Professional Advocacy.

After changing the authority structure between patients and physicians, the number of malpractice claims dropped by 75 percent. So I called Hickson to ask him about it. He graciously talked me through it.

Hickson studied only physicians at the time, but his work has implications for all medical providers.

He found that only a few doctors (6 percent) attracted almost half (40 percent) of malpractice suits and most (85 percent) of malpractice awards and settlements. He also found that these high-risk physicians thought their risk was average. They didn't know they were high risk, and they didn't know why. But Hickson did:

In our view, traditional peer review is ill-equipped to identify physician behaviors that dissatisfy their patients and place themselves at increased risk for unnecessary medical malpractice suits.[22]

On the phone, Hickson was affable, and assured me with a slow Tennessee drawl that I could call him anytime if I had more questions, putting me at ease. Then he laid out a common misunderstanding, "Patient satisfaction is not linked to lower malpractice risk," he said. "Patient dissatisfaction suggests a higher level of risk." Meaning patient dissatisfaction, rather than satisfaction, may be related to why patients sue their doctor.

Hickson found that when families sued their doctor, there was often poor doctor-family communication, and some families viewed their physicians as unconcerned. Coinciding with a bad outcome, this could lead to lawsuit. Rather than financial gain, families were largely interested in finding out what really happened. They wanted to know if things had

---

22 Gerald Hickson and James Pichert, "Identifying and Addressing Physicians at High Risk for Medical Malpractice Claims," In Press.

been done right, medically, and make sure what happened to their child wouldn't happen to anyone else.

"This changed my definition of professionalism," said Hickson.

Modern professionalism

In the 1970s, Hickson explained, our model of professionalism was purely competence based. If you knew your medicine, you were competent. It was focused, like a closed model of illness. But Hickson's findings have convinced him that we need a broader definition. For him, professionalism includes clearly communicating with patients, modeling respect (by including nurses as equal team members), and being available to patients. These form a foundation of trust between patient and provider.

Hickson went on to make sure I had not misunderstood,

The bane of my existence is a charming physician who makes families feel reassured, but is unskilled.

For him, skill is important, but it isn't enough. His definition of professionalism is holistic.

Giving patients a voice

Hickson created the Patient Advocacy Reporting System (PARS) to address the problem at Vanderbilt. It's a program in the Center for Patient and Professional Advocacy (CPPA), which he helped create. This system gives patients a voice. At Vanderbilt, if a patient has a complaint or concern, it's sent through the PARS office, where the staff catalogues the complaint. After a certain number of complaints, the CPPA office intervenes. The interventions fall into three levels, organized into a pyramid, because fewer physicians need escalated levels of intervention.

Level 1: Awareness intervention

At the first level, if physicians receive a certain number of complaints, they are visited. Their visitor is another physician, trained to objectively deliver the data to them, dispassionately. There is no other intervention, just information. Early in the development of the program, some physicians would throw the folder at the person delivering the data. But the message was, "I don't work where you work, and you will find a solution." Hickson reasoned that most physicians are capable, but haven't paused long enough to consider how they are perceived. The program assumed that most are able to self-correct. Failure to do so resulted in the next level of intervention.

Level 2: Authority intervention

Next they meet with an authority figure, one of the CPPA physicians trained to talk it out when the doctor failed to self-correct. Hickson calls it a "cup of coffee talk." Only a third of high-risk physicians need to move to this level. The physician is required to create a plan to address the complaints. Some physicians undergo communication training or personality-disorder screening. Others choose simply to lighten their clinical load.

Level 3: Disciplinary intervention

If the pattern persists despite the previous interventions, the provider is subject to disciplinary action, sometimes including termination. This is rare and has only occurred in about five of the approximately twelve hundred physicians working in the system.

Changes in the community

Hickson would be the first to point out that good things happening at his institution aren't only due to his program; there are other programs and factors at play.

That being said, since 1998, when the intervention began, Vanderbilt has seen a 75 percent drop in malpractice claims. After the CPPA got involved, patient complaints went down by about a third. Some physicians were resistant and others embraced the program. Those who embraced it saw a drop in patient complaints of 78 percent on average.

There was also a dark side to the program.

Although 60 percent of the high-risk physicians responded to a single meeting, one in five would ultimately leave the community. Hickson believes that these physicians are perpetually mobile, having difficulty settling in any community. They represent a group at significantly higher malpractice risk, and they are often new to their area.

Changing the authority structure changed the way that physicians and patients interacted at Vanderbilt. It began with a mild-mannered pediatrician listening to families who had arguably lost everything, and trying to shine insight into medical practice in his community.

Understanding that physicians did not recognize the limits of their ability to communicate, he simply created the CPPA, an unbiased third party with enough authority to speak clearly, and the perspective that they should only exercise that authority when necessary. High-risk physicians did not know their risk, but when confronted with it, they often self-corrected with rare recidivism.

Moving from a scientific model of competency to a more holistic view, Hickson was not met with the same level of resistance as Press. But as Hickson alluded to in his new definition of professionalism (Communication, Respect, Availability), it is more complicated than we once thought.

In an increasingly complex medical environment, we will find that the model of a lone-wolf provider making all the decisions with a hierarchy structure has an inferior risk profile to an older tribal approach. Given the complexity of the medical encounter, trading a hierarchy for a tribe makes our patients safer. Without our tribe, many of our efforts may be in vain.

Tribe versus hierarchy

In *Creativity Inc.* Pixar CEO Ed Catmull reveals one of the secrets of how his company created so many successful movies. He describes how the hierarchy structure worked well for top-down decision making, but not for the creative process. Pixar must do both tasks well. Like Odysseus, they have a complex mission requiring creative problem solving and systematically completing practical tasks with little error. In order to maximize creative productivity, he had to take the hierarchy of his company structure and turn it on its side into what is basically a tribal circle.

A hallmark of a healthy creative culture is that its people feel free to share ideas, opinions, and criticisms. Lack of candor, if unchecked, ultimately leads to dysfunctional environments.[23]

Within the tribe, ideas can float freely and members can innovate. The structure of the company creates fertile soil for what Pixar was trying to grow: great animated stories. Complexity was the challenge that full-length animated films had overcome in Pixar's explosion of success.

Complexity weaves through the ED. Each patient is unique with his or her own history and long medication list. We extract information, review records, perform procedures, and make high-stakes judgment calls, like admission or disposition.

This requires both creative thinking and checklist reliability. The importance of medical error demands that we have a tribal structure to facilitate both. Yes, a tribal structure is less efficient, and we need efficiency in the ED, but the more complicated medicine becomes, the more prone to error it is. As our practices become more futuristic, we make them safer by interacting more like a tribe. Each team member, RN, tech, or clerk, needs to be empowered so that if they see something, they will say something, and we will hear them.

Our tribal team in the ED is the crew of our ship. We sail in dangerous waters, and after we fix the holes in our ship (a.k.a. disruptive behaviors), we have to form an alliance with our crew. Providers can no longer go it alone with the increasing medical complexity in the modern era.

This is what Gerald Hickson meant by a new definition of professionalism. Competency is more than just the medicine. Today's providers must go further. Ruthlessly finding the holes in their ship and fixing them, and then pulling down the power hierarchy of the traditional medicine into a less fragile, more robust tribal structure. We are heroes. Will we see our tragic flaw before tragedy strikes?

We begin with the team.

---

23 Ed Catmull, *Creativity, Inc.: Overcoming the Unseen Forces That Stand in the Way of True Inspiration* (New York: Random House, 2014).

CHAPTER 12

THE ED TEAM

In many professions, what used to matter most were
abilities associated with the left side of the brain:
linear, sequential, spreadsheet kind of faculties.
Those still matter, but they're not enough.
—DANIEL H. PINK

Blind swiss cheese

Atul Gawande, Harvard surgeon and checklist researcher, created a safe-surgery checklist to address common errors before an operation began. He found that running the checklist with the OR team reduced complication rates from 11 percent to 7 percent, a massive reduction.[24]

One interesting aspect of that list was what appeared to be an unlikely critical step. Before the surgery starts, everyone states their name and role. How could this possibly help reduce surgical complications?

Gawande felt that by breaking down the barrier of hierarchy, members of the surgical team are more likely to identify dangerous circumstances. If they see any potential patient-safety issues, they speak up.

The more complex medicine becomes, the more our authority structure needs to move from hierarchy to tribe. Consider the swiss cheese model for patient safety. Each member of the medical team is

24 A. B. Haynes et al., "Safe Surgery Saves Lives Study Group. A Surgical Safety Checklist to Reduce Morbidity and Mortality in a Global Population," *New England Journal of Medicine* 360, no. 5 (2009): 491–9.

like a piece of swiss cheese. The holes in the cheese are unique to each individual's perspective and experience. Metaphorically, a patient-safety issue could go through one person's swiss cheese hole, but not through the next slice. Each of us is unique. Our holes are different. A problem is missed by the surgeon, but the scrub nurse picks it up, or the anesthesiologist. In this way, what makes us different makes our patients safer. But only if we do one critical step. We must give everyone the autonomy to speak up. This is a tribal-authority structure, not a hierarchy.

In actual cheese-making, the holes in swiss cheese are called eyes. The eyes are bubbles of gas created by the bacteria *Propionibacterium freudenreichii* that thrives in warmer media. (Swiss cheese is made at a higher temperature.) The bacteria do not act alone. During the process of milking the cows, tiny particles of hay fall into the milk and serve as nuclei for formation of the "eyes." This only happens if there is a human element to the cheese-making process. As modern milking technology has made the process more efficient, using machines in place of people, there are fewer holes. This is a major problem for swiss-cheese producers. The eyes make swiss cheese unique. Swiss cheese with no holes is called blind cheese.

Like in medicine, the ancient process had benefits that we didn't appreciate until the process was made machine efficient. Modern medical hierarchy is fast and efficient. The nurses, techs, and physicians each have a role. Having a tribe where everyone can provide input, unfortunately, makes the ED less efficient. But it's safer, and increased efficiency can come at a cost to safety. A tribal-authority structure helps us function as we have evolved, and will make us safer in a more complex environment. Cheese makers must sometimes resist new streamlined efficiencies in order to make quality cheese. To protect our patients, at times we must also resist. Newer is not always better.

Influence without power

Nurses and providers have a unique working relationship. Providers do not hire the nurses. We have completely separate authority structures. On the upside, that means that providers do not have to spend energy hiring and firing nursing staff (or vice versa), but having this unique structure creates unique problems. The main problem is how to work together well when we might have different ideas of what that means.

The history of nursing and physician practice happened in parallel. Physician history follows the tradition of Sir William Osler and the white coat. Medicine became increasingly evidence based and technology required a more tech-savvy practitioner.

Nursing has also undergone a dramatic change in the last fifty years. Nursing has become unionized. Training programs developed into schools, with Masters programs and now Doctoral programs. Nursing also publishes its own independent peer-reviewed literature in separate journals. The changes happening along different paths have created different cultures. Our differences make our patients safer. No blind swiss cheese here.

How do the cultures differ? Some might assert that provider culture is focused on evidence-based medicine and balancing autonomy with "best practices" for each disease entity. This protects our ability to practice the art of medicine while also agreeing that where the science is clear we should use the same therapy.

Nursing culture has focused on critical thinking or making sure that a patient's care makes sense. Some nursing education is focused on how to understand and follow treatment protocols, but there is also an emphasis on questioning why we do what we do.

Added to this is the power differential between provider and nurse. Providers evaluate patients, write orders, and prescribe therapy. Nurses do parallel evaluation, think critically, and carry out reasonable orders. Both provider and nursing education have limited emphasis on conflict resolution, leaving most conflicts between the two unaddressed.

Protecting working relationships

During our work day it's easy to become myopic and focus on logistical snags instead of our overall strategy. Nurses, other providers, and patients are all affected by your conduct in the ED. You have an opportunity to lead by example. When you sweat the small stuff you fail to lead effectively.

Critical provider priorities are as follows:

- Do no harm, practice mutual respect
- Open communication, tribal rather than top-down
- Intrinsically motivate others to do their best: autonomy, mastery, purpose

First, do no harm

As providers we take the oath passed down from Hippocrates thousands of years ago. We take it to mean that when caring for patients, avoid interventions that may cause more harm than good. While this edict is intended for patient care, it should also apply to our working relationships with nurses and other members of our team.

> *Never criticize, condemn, or complain.*
> —ANDREW CARNEGIE

The best advice ever given on this subject is written above. Many providers make the mistake of temporarily leaving their role of provider to pick up the role of nursing manager. This is a problem: providers have no expertise in nursing management.

Having a separate authority structure from the nursing staff allows us to focus on our own roles. If there are problems working together, it's best to give feedback to nursing managers. There may be exceptions where you have to give direct feedback, but you'll need to follow the tribal rule; if you see something (dangerous), say something (nonjudgmentally). Being critical is a hole in your boat. It's better to praise positive behavior.

Tribal structure

> *You can never win an argument.*
> —SOMEONE WHO SAVED A LOT OF TIME AND ENERGY

Hierarchies have strengths as well as weaknesses. We know who is in charge. When an order is given, it's clear what needs to happen next. Most hierarchies have recourse for inaccurate or bad orders.

Some situations lend themselves well to the model. The situation of a cardiac-arrest code works very well as a hierarchy. Action is needed, and there is a limited amount of creative heavy lifting. ACLS is an algorithm. But running a code in the ED is a relatively infrequent event, even in high-acuity EDs. Ironically, the crisis is relatively easy. Business as usual is harder to manage.

Fortunately for providers, and our job security, most patients' illnesses are complex and poorly managed by an algorithm. For the newly presenting patient, the team gets the facts straight: complaint, history, meds, etc. Then, we use creative brain circuits to form a differential diagnosis. Next, we employ divergent thinking to imagine different possibilities for treatment and to critically consider risks and benefits. Experienced providers consider the quality of the information available and whether or not the patient is really harboring a fatal disease dressed up as a benign complaint. If the diagnosis becomes clear after this, or with testing, then the team uses convergent thinking to select the appropriate treatment. Clinical uncertainty requires thinking about other possible scenarios and consequences of missing the diagnosis, then how likely they are, and how to minimize the patient's risk; for example, close follow up, admission for observation. It's complicated. And which structure is least suited for this complex task? Hierarchy.

Top-down structure limits creative thinking to the upper levels. Team members in the remainder of the structure wait for orders rather than being actively recruited to think creatively about the problem. Efficiency is a value of the hierarchy, and members may not want to sacrifice the system's efficiency for what might seem a minor safety issue. More efficient teams become more like blind cheese as their process is refined.

Like Pixar, we need all the creative and divergent thinking we can get, but if we don't ask for help, we won't get any. Evolving in tribes, we are already wired to be social contributing members of a small tribe at work; just look at all the unsolicited advice ("help") we already get. Having the opportunity to contribute stimulates the reward part of our brains and helps us feel valued. When your nursing teammates are invested in the process, they feel ownership. When you ask for their help, they understand you value their expertise.

The converse is also true. When we fail to work as a team, patient care suffers. Patients are triaged, then intake is done by the nurse. The nurse takes a history and writes (or "hides") it in the chart, where it will be lost forever, never to be found. The patient continues to wait. Then you enter. Introducing yourself, you ask the patient to repeat their history, which often comes off as unprofessional and sloppy. No one likes to repeat themselves. *No one* likes to repeat themselves. The history you take is in parallel with what the nurse got from the patient, and there is no function designed to reconcile these two attempts to gather information. Nurses take a history that, because it is often not reviewed by the provider, may never impact patient care, and this does not encourage their active involvement. Our crew is not engaged. Gawande engaged his team, as discussed earlier, with his Safe-Surgery Checklist. Step...ONE:

- *Confirm all team members have introduced themselves by name and role.*

The message to nurses: you have a role, you are responsible for the patient and their outcome, and you are allowed to speak, even during surgery. I am not suggesting that we have a formal step for each patient where the nurse and the provider touch base, but would that be so bad?

The communication in the ED must mimic that of Pixar, tribal in structure, so that information and ideas can flow unhindered. Will efficiency suffer? Perhaps. But there is uncaptured value in creative thinking and breaking down barriers for patient safety. That value comes from team communication. Without it efficiency improves, but like swiss cheese without eyes, we risk overlooking key details.

Humans were selected to develop in tribes, leaving us with biases and heuristics that trip us when we try to navigate complexity. We are not machines. As our world becomes more complex, we may find that, at least in the ED, reverting back to a more tribal way of thinking, ironically, protects us and our patients. Patients are safer when we communicate more informally and shed the medical hierarchy.

Intrinsic motivation

A lot of white-collar work requires less of the routine, rule-based, what we might call algorithmic set of capabilities, and more of the harder-to-outsource, harder-to-automate, non-routine, creative, juristic—as the scholars call it—abilities.
—DANIEL H. PINK

Sitting around on a night shift with nothing to do, I listened to the nurses talk about hospital projects for patient satisfaction. These nurses were in their sixties and nearing retirement. They had long memories. There were programs with gimmicks, touchy feely stuff. Then there were added questions to the intake questions. These ranged from the sensible screen, "Are you safe at home?" to the misguided jargonist, "What are your expectations for your ED visit?" Listening to their comic list, it was obvious that top-down change just doesn't work. It's not always tyranny, but it is oppressive.

"It's a fear-based culture," said Kathy Bartholomew, RN, author of *Speak Your Truth: Proven Strategies for Effective Nurse-Physician Communication.* Bartholomew, originally interested in the civil rights movement, transitioned from her nursing career to author and speaker, frustrated by the failures of our hospital culture. She describes an unwritten hierarchy that no one talks about, the barrier to open communication. For her, it's not only the changes in policy dictated to nursing staff by administration, but also the tolerance of providers' disruptive behavior.

"Our greatest strength is our greatest weakness. We tell ourselves stories to justify behavior: they're tired or recently divorced. We are grateful we are not the worst one in the room." Nurses tolerate disruptive behavior of physicians, which is also ignored by the administration. Instead of changing the power structure, Bartholomew instead sees more referendums of top-down quality initiatives.

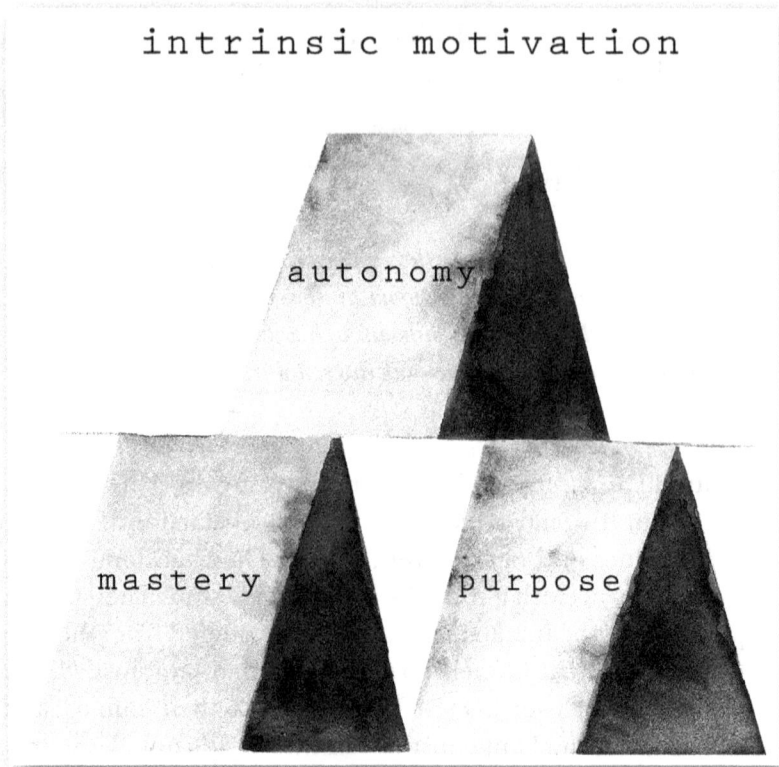

intrinsic motivation

autonomy

mastery   purpose

Following the above, a discussion about motivation rings false. Instead, inclusion should be our goal. Motivation is a by-product. The anatomy of an authentically motivating task is described by Daniel Pink in his book *Drive*. Pink outlines the structure as a triad: purpose, mastery, and autonomy.

Purpose

Purpose refers to our tendency to be motivated to accomplish things that really matter to us. No one wants to rearrange chairs on the deck of the Titanic. It's moot. But when we recognize that we have a unique ability to make a difference, it gives us purpose. Purpose drives us to work, and health care is filled with purpose. Forcing a mandated pointless task kills motivation, because the purpose is lost.

Mastery

Mastery describes our need for flow; the feeling that we are immersed in our task and time flies by while we watch ourselves work. Pink points out that we need a relatively difficult task in order to reach the flow state. No one gets excited about tic-tac-toe. We have a draw. Another draw. For authentic motivation, we need chess. We need critical care.

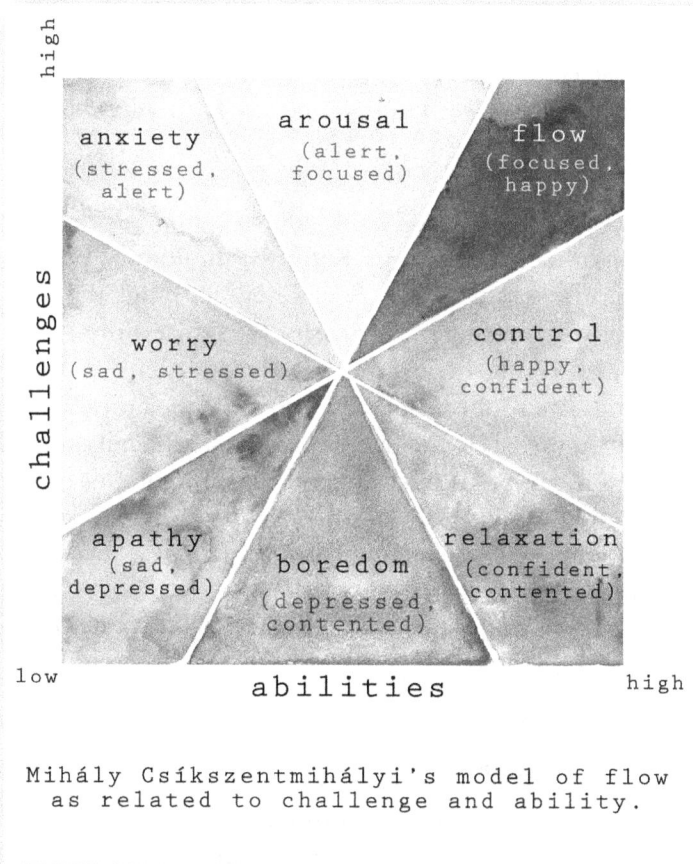

Mihály Csíkszentmihályi's model of flow as related to challenge and ability.

Autonomy

Autonomy, our ability to do our work the way we want, is both the foundation of intrinsic motivation and the part cut out by hierarchies.

Modern nursing builds a foundation of basic science, critical thinking, and clinical skills. Nursing professionals are too highly skilled to feel motivated by even complex emergency care if providers deny them autonomy. Experience only makes the price of this precious commodity go up. Autonomy is so important to professional satisfaction that author Cal Newport, when describing Daniel Pink's Triad, calls it the "Dream Job Elixir."

> *Giving people more control over what they do and how they do it increases their happiness, engagement, and sense of fulfillment.*[25]

Genuine interest

"Knowing each-other's stories," as Kathy Bartholomew puts it, means taking genuine interest in others. Social contact pings the reward centers of our brains. We quickly and easily recognize false interest. This counterfeit social capital is poisonous. It is vital that we take genuine interest in building rapport with our nursing colleagues. Contact with other providers in the ED is relatively minimal. Physicians and advanced practice providers are often busy and working in parallel play like children busy in the sandbox. Maintaining your working relationships with your real colleagues, your nurses, takes energy and investment. We get the most return on this investment by focusing on protecting autonomy, engaging in open communication, and being genuinely interested in our teammates.

The power of "sure" and decision fatigue

There is an easy way to protect autonomy. During the course of our ED shift, providers suffer from what researchers call decision fatigue. At the beginning of your shift, you have high energy, perhaps full of empathy and ready to make a difference. You throw yourself into your work, but find that around hour four you begin to fatigue; physically and emotionally.

---

25 Cal Newport, *So Good They Can't Ignore You: Why Skills Trump Passion in the Quest for Work You Love* (New York: Grand Central, 2012).

The specifics of each case you encounter begin to blur, and sometimes you begin to have trouble doing the labor of caring for your patients. Some of this labor is emotional caring, but most of it consists of doing basic things well each time: listening, examining, and carefully making decisions. There is a lot of responsibility, and you need to unload.

An easy way to do this is by allowing your colleagues to help protect your decision-making capacity, which generally fatigues reliably after a certain amount of work. You can do this by having them participate in making decisions. The next time your nursing or ED tech colleagues come to you with a suggestion, find a way to say "sure." Delegating decisions appropriately to your seasoned partners protects your cognitive reserves, and avoids sabotaging team motivation by micromanaging everyone.

When you depend on your team to help make decisions it does not go unnoticed. They should be accountable, but most will welcome the ability to help customize care.

Public appreciation, private feedback

Finally, remember to show sincere appreciation in public and give constructive feedback in private. Have your mood set the emotional tone for the department, positively managing morale when the going gets tough. Complaining leaders hurt morale, and when we complain about others, we sabotage social capital with everyone involved.

Changing your own habits is hard, but those who don't adapt will go extinct.

CHAPTER 13

CONVEYING VALUE TO SUPERVISING PHYSICIANS AND SPECIALISTS

Successful interactions with physician supervisors

Advanced practice providers in the Emergency Department have a uniquely challenging task. Their job involves a lot of people. They evaluate patients, identify emergencies (while conveying value to their patients and teams), while also following the guidelines of their attending physicians. Being successful favors experience, expertise, and a pound of luck.

If that wasn't enough, many providers work with multiple attending physicians each day. Shifting from one style to the next as the attending changes, while maintaining rapport and productivity are, to say the least, challenging.

Working with your attending physicians will be less difficult when you know what they want from you. Typically, what they want falls into three models based on the stage of your relationship. We will call the stages early, familiar, and expert working relationships.

Early working relationships

Regardless of experience level, the early period is marked by earning and keeping trust for your clinical skills. Can you show that you can take a reliable history? Patient's stories have a tendency to change during an encounter, so the game is unfair to begin with, but how accurate is the history you get? Is your physical exam reproducible?

Studies find that statistical inter-rater reliability for the physician exam is poor, even between physicians. It's not as dependable as an EKG or someone's hemoglobin level. Vital signs also have some variation, but they can be more reliably reproduced. Much of the reproducibility of the history and physical exam comes from having an understanding of how your attending physicians describe their patients. Seeing patients together helps, but it takes time to learn their styles.

Next is the plan of care. You must decide on a plan that your supervising physician would find agreeable. Each physician has different practice habits. While this clinical variation can be frustrating, the easiest way to learn the habits of supervising physicians is to read their dictations or other medical records. Nurses can also be a helpful source of information, and nothing is better than having frank discussions about their view for best practice for common presenting complaints. How do they feel pneumonia is best treated? What do they feel makes a patient with chest pain high risk?

To build this part of the relationship smoothly, it helps to make time for a discussion about your attending physicians' preferences and what they view as best practices. Building a common vocabulary helps you communicate effectively. When presenting patients, it's important to follow a structure that, at first, gives a fair amount of clinical detail. It should also be structured to help the attending physician understand the patient's presentation. With time the presentation can be streamlined.

Presenting patients to attending physicians

The purpose of the presentation is to give relevant clinical information that helps your attending decide on a treatment plan. In the early working relationship, more detail should be included to build trust and make your attending physician feel comfortable with your thoroughness. Some providers make the mistake of regurgitating all the information as it was received from the patient, like recording the interview and playing it back. This is a waste of time and can be worse than if the physician had done the entire encounter by themselves.

Constructing the oral presentation for emergency medicine starts with a solid encounter. First, the provider sits down with the patient and builds rapport to get things started on the right foot. Listening without interrupting empties patients' working memory and helps them feel heard so they can concentrate on other things, like the listening skills of their provider. Asking a few key questions about patients' stories and what you have read about their background helps fill in the gaps. Then, during your physical exam, explain to them what we are looking for, and what you see.

After leaving the room, switch your mental mode from information gathering to creative. Create your differential diagnosis, including several key life-threatening possibilities (worst-first), and imagine how the information you have gathered helps sort out the possible diagnoses.

Then, before presenting, you need to work backward. Start with what you think is wrong, your working diagnosis. Include two others to keep your mind open, then organize your information to show how your reached that diagnosis, and why it's not other life-threatening conditions.

Here's the key: Instead of giving a verbal summary of the patient's story, organize the information. Synthesize an argument. Begin with your working diagnosis and go back through the history and physical to list the basic elements that support or refute it. This will structure your plan.

Here's an example:

Bad presentation

> *Sixty-seven-year-old female came to the ED after she was cooking, and feeling angry because her husband was not listening to her, she asked him to leave but then felt pain in her chest that she cannot describe. It came with a feeling of sweatiness, and she didn't want to call 911 because she was baking, but last time this happened she had to have a stent for her heart attack, and they told her she had a heart murmur, which I hear. She also has a rash on her legs and a healing cut on her left arm from last week. She doesn't really want to stay in the hospital, but thinks she may have to because she passed out.*

The main problem with this presentation is the lack of organization. When you list the symptoms, chest pain, syncope, diaphoresis, and include a history of heart disease with coronary stenting, it sounds high risk. But woven in with the patient's narrative it becomes harder to follow. Part of the physical exam is also included in the history. This is distracting because it doesn't follow the way most physicians process the information: symptoms, past medical history, medications, then physical exam and data. When things are out of order, or blended, the story becomes unclear.

Better presentation

Sixty-seven-year-old female with history of CAD and stenting presents with an episode of left precordial pressure for fifteen minutes while cooking and arguing with her spouse. The chest pain was associated with diaphoresis but no shortness of breath, or history of pulmonary embolism. Pain was similar to previous MI, but has resolved. On Review of Systems the patient described a syncopal episode last week when standing to walk to the bathroom, she fell and was evaluated in the ED with a small laceration, then discharged after being watched overnight. Physical Exam shows normal vital signs except a BP of 167/78 and a previously described systolic murmur, but no signs of heart failure or pneumonia. She told me she prefers not to stay in the hospital but her health is her priority, so she'll stay if she has to.

It's clear and actionable; the patient needs to be admitted to the hospital.

Optimal communication

Bad presentations are hard to follow and important details are not easy to hear. This makes it harder to sort the patient into a category that helps create a good plan. After listening, the attending physicians will need to organize the information themselves and likely talk to the patient in greater detail. It's hard to trust a disorganized presentation because it creates more work for everyone or, worse, causes more testing for the patient and risk of complications. Our second presentation has a differential in mind: myocardial infarction (history of cardiac stents), pulmonary embolism (dyspnea and no previous embolism), and pneumonia. Next the provider might list their working differential and plan.

Changing the discussion to separately describe the syncopal episode allows the team to truncate its discussion. We know it is unrelated to today's complaint, but now understand the patient's healing laceration, and also that a recent hospitalization puts the patient at higher risk of pulmonary embolism.

There is labor involved to create a simple picture of complex circumstances:

> *[S]implicity is not so simple to attain. Steve Jobs figured out*
> *that "you have to work hard to get your thinking clean to*
> *make it simple." The Arabs have an expression for trenchant*
> *prose: no skill to understand it, mastery to write it.*[26]
> —Nassim Taleb

Familiar working relationships
Growth of trust strengthens our efficiency as a team. In early working relationships it is often helpful to evaluate and examine patients together. Simultaneous evaluation builds a common vocabulary. A face-to-face evaluation of every patient is less necessary over time. Hence, when things don't fit the pattern, it is important for the advanced practice providers to ask their attending physicians to have a look. This protects the patient and continues to build the relationship. Eventually, the practice patterns will become routine enough to move to an expert working relationship, usually after several years of close work with an attending physician.

Conveying value to consultants
Interactions with specialists in the ED can either be a high-powered fulcrum for conveying your true value to your group, or a total disaster.

---

26 Taleb, *AntiFragile, Things That Gain From Disorder.*

Many specialists feel that they want their ED staff to be highly specific and accurate when we need to call them. While this is important, we also need to be highly sensitive, missing nothing. It feels heroic to make a great diagnosis or save, but what our patients really need is for us to do the simple things well. Then do them well repeatedly, very well, over and over again, in a way that can be relied upon. The problem is reliable isn't very sexy.

Limited time speaking with our specialist colleagues means higher risk for misunderstandings and false impressions. Presentations need to be refined and brief. Take time before contacting the specialist to get organized, and so your presentation can shine.

The ED is a fishbowl; everyone can see what you do in practice. Rocking the boat makes everyone uncomfortable. Unfortunately, the perspective of the specialist often doesn't take into account our unique challenges in the ED: patient flow, resource management, and the accountability that comes from being open to any patient, at any time. They don't work in the ED, so most don't understand.

Action-focused approach for specialist interaction

In order to optimize your interaction, it's best to lead with exactly what you want your specialists to do for each patient. Convey enough information to adequately build the context, and respect their time on the phone.

We generally call specialists for one of three reasons:

1. To perform a procedure such as an appendectomy, or endoscopy.
2. To co-manage a complex patient, for example pregnant trauma patients.
3. To provide expert advice or consultation on a patient for the ED over the phone.

Your presentation should be action oriented. Which of the three do you need them to do? For example, for all the specialist knows you could be asking for advice on the case, or perhaps to do surgery. Maybe you want the specialist to admit the patient, or just be aware that the patient is on a hospitalist service, and take a look in the morning. Specialists will hear more relevant details if they know what you expect them to do from the outset.

It is important to give all the information they need to make the decision that you want them to make. It helps to know the decision ahead of time, for example, an appendectomy for appendicitis. In this case, you want to give the pertinent history, any other important information (such as whether the patient NPO), and a focused physical exam. Extra information will just serve to confuse and distract, unless there are patient-safety concerns.

Concretely, a patient comes in, gets testing done, and you feel the patient needs an appendectomy. Begin the conversation, "I have a patient who I feel needs an appendectomy." This way the action is clear, and there is no vague notion that you may actually want to discharge the patient to be seen in clinic or that you're unclear of the diagnosis. Your intentions and expectations are clear from the outset. Then you give other pertinent information once your intentions are clear.

"I have a patient who needs an appendectomy, and who presented with right-lower quadrant pain for two days with tenderness at McBurney's point, and a CT scan that shows appendicitis." At this point you might give the surgeon other information, but first you are focusing the conversation by stripping down the information and organizing it. Next, answer any questions and then verbalize the plan to make sure you are both clear.

From the specialist's perspective, you are an outsider. It is unfair for you to be treated like this, but you must earn trust. No one deserves to be mistreated, but sometimes it's not just the patient who is having a bad day.

Harbor no ill will against grumpy consultants, and you may win them over. Bitterness is poisonous. Don't fall into the trap. If the situation is abusive, contact a third party, documenting facts rather than inflammatory details. Managing your more difficult colleagues often requires better organization before you call them. Sometimes it's necessary to involve your attending physician, so you can stay focused on the patient.

If you have a disagreement, and admission or intervention is what you feel is necessary, then reiterate your reasons. But remember that you cannot force anyone to do anything, even if you are the chair of the hospital board. You will have to compromise at times, and at that point, you must always involve your attending physician. Then it's best to discuss with the patient that there are gray areas and more than one method in patient care. Always speak positively about your specialist consultants to your patients.

CHAPTER 14

CUSTOMER-SERVICE RESCUE

Recognition of the cultural differences between patient and provider will help improve patients' experiences. Using a checklist will help meet nonmedical needs and significantly decrease the frequency of negative interactions. But no matter what you do, you cannot make all the people happy all the time.

Patients understand that their provider is not perfect. Some might fall into the trap of the fundamental attribution error, as we all do, and make a judgment about their provider's character that will be hard to overcome. Unfortunately, of all the patients who have some level of dissatisfaction with their visit, few will complain. Those who do have given us a gift.

Given a second chance

Patients who complain during their ED visit give the team a chance to, first, recognize what happened, and then to start customer-service rescue. Sometimes what upsets patients can be a legitimate safety hazard: lack of communication, disruptive behavior, or bloody needles on the floor. Then their complaint will make your ED a safer place for other patients and decrease risk to everyone. Those who telegraph their unhappiness are often open to discussing it.

Customer-service rescue starts with careful listening. The provider should be seated to decrease the power-distance index, and to show respect. Often patients and their families are angry, and this anger is directed at the provider. It's difficult not to take it personally, but re-member that the cognitive processes that judge competency are auto-matic. They are, by definition, snap judgments. There is no way they can possibly know if you are competent. So it's not personal, it's bias. Try to let it roll off your back.

The mountain of anger

The mountain of anger is a concept used to train people who take com-plaints for a living. (If you are ever frustrated hearing the occasional complaint, just be thankful you don't do it full time.) When people begin to vent anger, they access the part of their brain where the in-formation is stored, and the emotion anger boils up with it. Just like remembering a pleasant memory brings the sunshine of nostalgia, nega-tive memories come with negative emotions. It is critical that the listener lets them completely vent their complaint. Much of the information may be unfair, untrue, or irrelevant. It doesn't matter. And the patients know that not all the accusations are fair. But the important task at this time is to let patients or family members vent completely to get to the top of the mountain of anger.

If they are interrupted, or you add little corrections to their com-plaints, even clarifications, they get knocked down the mountain and need to climb it again. It will take longer, and they will get more upset. As a professional, much of what we do involves emotional labor. It can be every bit as difficult as physical labor. Let your patients get to the top of the mountain of anger without interrupting their climb.

Apology

Then you must apologize. It may not be your fault. It may not be any-one's fault. The complaint might not even be legitimate. But in human conflict, apology is the antidote. Listen to the complaint, don't take it personally (read: stay calm), and apologize.

After an apology, patients and their families will want to know a brief plan for how you will make sure this doesn't happen to someone else. Usually it is as simple as: we will document and review this issue. Most complaints are documented and reviewed by the quality improvement or medical staff departments of the hospital. Reassure the patient that this is your plan, so this issue will not happen to another person.

Consequences of ignoring complaints

Complaints that are not voiced in the ED are sent on to the hospital administration. Often another person will need to have the same conversation with the patient, and then with you. Some complaints will require other meetings, additional conversations, and additional consequences. The true cost of a complaint is a significant amount of time and money lost. And as noted earlier, complaints increase risk of malpractice lawsuit.

Customer-service rescue helps decrease risk because in order to complain it requires a certain amount of emotional energy, more for some people than others. When we begin the process in the ED, sometimes that can defuse the situation. The complaint might stop right there, without further action. That is why most risk managers recommend apology for medical errors by the provider, and why customer-service rescue decreases risk of malpractice suit.

Remember that everyone has a unique perspective and that patients help us when they complain in the ED instead of waiting to do it later. Shoulder the load and do the emotional labor of customer-service rescue. Skill in this area will make you valuable and difficult to replace. Your hard work will not go unnoticed and you will convey value to your peers. Also, remember that your perspective is biased by the fundamental attribution error, too. The patient is stuck in the hardest of circumstances. If he or she needs to vent, be empathetic.

CHAPTER 15

FINAL THOUGHTS

Letter to my younger self.

Dear Friend,

I want you to know a few things that will make life easier for you and your patients.

I'll begin by telling you that there is a big difference between patient culture and medical culture, and there will be misunderstandings.

Trying the same strategies harder won't bridge this gap, you have to adopt a different approach, but if something doesn't work for you, forget it, try something else that feels authentic. Patients can tell, and they value your authenticity.

When you enter a room and meet another person, you need to respect the history of human evolution; it's a sacred moment and demands what we might call a ritual: eyes, kindness, and time.

Your medical colleagues will judge your competency one way, but your patients will rely on how well you communicate. When things don't seem to be going well, you need to return to this simple truth. Communicate clearly, respectfully, keep patients informed, and have the humility to know your closed model of illness isn't the only way to see things.

Realize that different parts of the ED encounter have different weights in each patient's experience, invest time in the beginning and end of the encounter, and consider a call after the visit. Make the hardest part of each visit a little easier. Plan in a patient-centered way.

Know that you cannot achieve perfect patient satisfaction, but that a better experience of care relieves suffering. Anxious patients suffer. They are unsure of their future. Comfort them.

Know that if you commit to doing it right each time, it may not feel like you're improving, but you are. Trust the process.

Remember that what you do matters. Now, how will *you* do it?

APPENDIX

HEURISTICS THAT BLIND THE MEDICAL MIND

Note to the reader: When I wrote this chapter, about how heuristics affect medical decision making, it didn't fit well into the preceding text. In my own practice, it has been helpful to know when I might be biased, so I included the chapter here as an appendix. You may also enjoy reading Pat Croskerry's paper on the subject, available free online:

Croskerry P. The importance of cognitive errors in diagnosis and strategies to minimize them. Acad Med. 2003 Aug;78(8):775–80. Peter Wason's puzzle is also fascinating, and a great way to ruin a dinner party.

It's date night. My wife and I are brought downstairs, in a building outside town, with two other couples. The dark room has a single light hanging, dimly. There are no windows. We sit around a black desk in plastic chairs, facing each other.

"You will be given three problems to solve in the next sixty minutes," says our hostess. She seems bored, and this is her memorized intro.

"If you succeed, the door will unlock, and you may leave. If not, then we will release the zombies."

Looking for something novel and fun on date night, we signed up for an evening with a few of our friends at the Puzzle Room. Some of their clients are friends who signed up together, although you can choose to be grouped with strangers, too. When you sign up, you can also choose different scenarios. We picked zombies. What could be better than zombies? Nothing.

The first problem we get is interactive. We are given a series of numbers that follow a rule. They are 2, 4, 8. Then we are instructed that we cannot ask about the rule. Instead we may give our own series of three numbers in order to try to figure out the rule. Our guide can only reply yes, if the sequence follows the mystery rule, or no, if it doesn't. Then, when we think we know the rule, we write it down and seal it in an envelope that is dropped into a slot. Remember, we are locked in. There is only one envelope, so we only get one guess, and we have to get it right before we can move on to the next puzzle. The zombies probably won't go to bed hungry.

So I start. "Ten, twenty, forty?"

"Yes, it follows the rule."

Then my wife says, "Fifty, one hundred, two hundred?"

Yes. So we write down the rule, number doubles each time, and toss it in the slot, smiling. Let's get to the hard stuff, we think.

"Your answer was incorrect," says our guide, without a smile. "We will now release the zombies."

In 1999, the Institute of Medicine put out a report estimating that ninety-eight thousand Americans die as a result of medical errors. The report was heavily criticized and later studies took a more careful look into the impact of medical errors on clinical outcomes. Although the statistic, ninety-eight thousand preventable deaths, is almost certainly as preposterous as it sounds, other studies have reliably found that medical errors happen at a rate of approximately 10–15 percent. This is based on diagnosis prior to death compared to diagnosis on autopsy.[27][28]

27 E. Tejerina, et al., "Clinical Diagnoses and Autopsy Findings: Discrepancies in Critically Ill Patients," *Crit Care Med* 40, no. 3 (2012): 842–6.

28 K. G. Shojania, E. C. Burton, K. M. McDonald, and L. Goldman, "Changes in Rates of Autopsy Detected Diagnostic Errors over Time," *JAMA* 289 (2003): 2849–56.

Premortem compared to postmortem, and how often we get it right.

With the introduction of heuristics to clinical medicine, we now realize that many errors can be attributed to cognitive bias by clinicians.

Cognitive errors, also called heuristics, stem from the same ancient brain origins in medical providers as they do in everyone else. The automatic system, or system one, works effortlessly and instantly to recognize patterns and evaluate patients, while our deliberate system two takes a back seat. In evaluating patients, most of the information acquisition is in our history taking, which lends well to our automatic system, evolved for interpersonal interaction in tribes. Researchers studying medical decision making suggest that we often use "dual processing," activating both the deliberate, analytical *system two* and the automatic *system one*, interactively. Biases come when we rely too much on our lightning-fast automatic system, evolved for tribal living and poorly adapted to complex decision making.

Clinical cognitive biases fall into the same three categories as non-clinical ones: tendency toward confirmation (confirmation bias), ease of memorial retrieval (availability heuristic), and recognizing false patterns (representativeness). Applying these to different clinical scenarios has led to the naming of numerous medical diagnostic traps specific to different situations, and with significant overlap.

Arguably, the three most important have been named: *anchoring bias*, *base-rate neglect*, and *visceral bias*. Each of these is a product of a different mismatch of our cognitive tendencies to the complex decisions we make in medicine each shift. The first stems from our tendency toward confirmation.

Meanwhile, back in the dank dungeon on date night, I was wondering if we could order cocktails. We were waiting for our time to run out so we could be devoured by zombies. If I'm going to be condemned to an eternity of mindless hunger for human flesh, I might have one last Manhattan. Our hostess ignored my question about what kind of bourbon they stock and continued her memorized lines:

"Before we release the zombies, you have one last chance to get out of here alive." She started describing our next puzzle without taking a drink order, but none of us had any idea what the real answer was on the first number-sequence question.

It turns out that the number sequence problem was borrowed from a British psychologist, Peter Wason, who, in addition to coining the phrase confirmation bias, also created a series of experiments to demonstrate our tendency toward confirmation.[29] His sequence was actually 2-4-6, and he found that people largely used confirmatory questions when they listed numbers to see what the rule might be. That is, they would give a sequence that they thought would work. When it worked, they felt they were right.

What they should have done was to test their hypothesis. Maybe the answer was that the numbers double? So subjects would try 10-20-40, and it would work. Maybe the rule was that the number would follow the rule n + 2? So they would try 106-108-110, and it would work, confirming their suspicion. Although this was not a difficult sequence, the answer was "any increasing sequence of numbers," and only six of the original twenty-nine subjects got the answer right on the first try. Many never figured it out and got eaten by zombies.

Anchoring bias

Anchoring bias is the tendency to either get stuck on one diagnosis or to give a suggested diagnosis more weight despite having inadequate evidence to support it. This is part of everyday experience in medicine, and has also been demonstrated experimentally.[30] Take the example of a patient with chest pain and EKG changes sent from cardiology clinic with a concern for cardiac ischemia. The tests show normal cardiac enzymes, and the patient is admitted as an acute coronary syndrome only to die from a pulmonary embolism. Atypical pulmonary emboli are infrequent but not rare, but the diagnosis of angina had inertia after it was

---

29 P. C. Wason, "On the Failure to Eliminate Hypotheses in a Cognitive Task," *Quarterly Journal of Experimental Psychology* 12 (1960): 129–40.

30 V. R. LeBlanc, G. R. Norman, and L. R. Brooks, "Effect of a Diagnostic Suggestion on Diagnostic Accuracy and Identification of Clinical Features," *Acad Med* 76 (2001): S18–20.

suggested by the clinic. The ED provider was anchored, and failed to give consideration to other causes of chest pain.

The provider's tendency toward confirmation is a bug in the same software that kept Wason's number-sequence subjects from asking the right questions. Namely, what should I ask to disprove my hypothesis. Does 3-2-1 work? No? Why is that? Instead most subjects, myself included, tend to seek data to confirm the suspicions of our automatic system. Although this works fast and efficiently with most decisions, it will get you eaten by zombies on date night.

I would like to tell you that the next bias, base-rate neglect, came up during date night, too, but it didn't. It came up on a drive home from vacation with my family when I was listening to *Nudge*, a book by Richard Thaler who, after working with behavioral economist Daniel Kahneman, cameoed for himself in the movie *The Big Short*. Kahneman and Thaler also advise a mutual fund company together, based on behavioral economics.

In *Nudge*, Thaler notes that most people suppose incorrectly that more people die each year from homicide than suicide. They don't. My wife and I also thought that death from homicide had to be way more common, and we were shocked, so much that we stared at each other open mouthed. I veered into the left lane and we almost hit a police car.

Traffic accidents kill many more people than homicide, but after I almost hit the police car I was sure my wife was going to kill me.

Base-rate neglect

Base-rate neglect is the failure of clinicians to accurately estimate prevalence, like homicide, or death by collision with a police car. Our automatic systems prefer to use information that is more easily retrieved from our memories. Whatever comes to mind easier seems more likely.[31] Drowning is more prevalent than shark attack, and pneumonia kills more people than West Nile Virus. However, despite this, when outbreaks of illnesses such as West Nile are reported in the media, testing increases among clinicians, even in areas of the country where the virus is unlikely to be found.

31 S. Lichtenstein, P. Slovic, B. Fischhoff, M. Layman, and B. Combs, "Judged Frequency of Lethal Events,"
Journal of Experimental Psychology: Human 4, no. 6 (1978): 551–78.

It is said that when you hear hoofbeats, think horse, not zebra. The cognitive error is from the same maladaptive cognitive systems that cause us to misjudge competency in areas where we lack expertise. We can't easily access the information required to make a sound judgment, so we make a substitution, and a quick estimate that is rarely accurate. Unfortunately, because the cognitive system is automatic, it is subconscious so we are often unaware of our bias.

Visceral bias

Visceral Bias, a consequence of our unbridled automatic system, blinds us because of our tendency to over rely on our first impression of the patient's condition. Coupled with our tendency toward confirmation, clinicians fail to consider other diagnoses, or discordant data. Just like our patients, who sometimes misjudge providers based on first impressions, we also make a snap judgment. Influenced by our impression, we could fail to make the right diagnosis if we don't make a conscious effort to engage our deliberate system, and think analytically.

Currently there is little proven strategy for overcoming cognitive bias in clinical decision making. Pulling the mask seems to help. It is understanding that we need to ask questions to disprove our impressions, at least in the number-sequence problem. Other researchers recommend what they call "operationalized reflection" or systematic decision making. We benefit by deliberately engaging our deliberate system.

Clinical decision rules can be used to add analytical double checks to our clinical gestalt. Many electronic medical records now have what are known as "forcing functions," steps in the ordering and discharge process designed to make the provider double-check clinical details. One example is electronic medical records that flag abnormal vital signs at the time of discharge, requiring the provider to check off on a patient's fever that may have otherwise gone unnoticed.

Unfortunately, after the first day of using the program, our automatic system already begins to click through without looking. The truth is, we will always have some degree of bias, and we need to be aware that it can affect our patients' care.

THE BRIDGE DISCUSSION QUESTIONS

Part I

1. Why did you choose medicine?
2. What are the parts of practicing medicine that you love and why?
3. What aspect of practicing medicine do you dread? Why?
4. What are some reasons providers may have difficulty connecting with their patients?
5. Describe what is meant by nonmedical needs of emergency patients.
6. What is the fundamental attribution error?
7. What is the halo effect?
8. Describe competency bias.
9. Discuss an experience in your life that was disproportionally affected by the end of the experience.
10. What is emotional concretization?

Part II

1. Build a checklist for a laceration repair including key steps so that it is done right every time.
2. What is acuity dissonance? Have you experienced it and can you tell the story?
3. Explain the vertical-horizontal framework.

4. Give three examples of how you might venerate members of your team to your patients in the ED.

5. What do you do for fun? How does it make you feel to talk about it with others?

6. To practice patient teaching, give a short one-minute talk giving patient information on a common topic i.e. influenza, recovery from ankle fracture, return precautions for possible pediatric appendicitis, etc...

7. Create your own checklist for an ED encounter.

Part III

1. Why do we tolerate verbal abuse in medicine?

2. Explain the swiss cheese model of patient safety.

3. With regards to intrinsic motivation, explain what is meant by autonomy, mastery, and purpose.

4. What is meant by flow and what conditions are required to achieve it? When have you experienced it in your life? How could you experience it at work?

5. Describe your approach to patient presentations to attending physicians or consultants.

6. What is meant by the mountain of anger?

7. Describe anchoring bias?

8. Give an example of how you have been biased by base-rate neglect.

ACKNOWLEDGMENTS

This book was the culmination of efforts from multiple people. The most central to the project was, obviously, Irwin Press, who has spent most of his professional life advocating for patient-centered emergency medicine. Gerald Hickson was also tremendously helpful and generous with his time. Dan Batson kindly allowed me to ask him about his work, as he has allowed countless others over the last fifty or so years. Kathy Bartholomew was gracious enough to discuss the material with me and give me her considerable insight. Thanks to my wife, Kelly, who tolerated my countless hours of seclusion in my dark study while she wrangled our boys. She is an amazing woman: tolerant, nurturing, and brilliant. Joanna Bartlett helped me develop the book after my first few initial drafts. She was patient and kind. I would also be remised not to thank my colleagues in the ED, Eric Spencer and Harry Kleiner, who continue to make each work day better and constantly inspire me to be a better doctor. Also Deborah Herman, who provided feedback on the manuscript and who works hard every day for our patients. To the patients we sometimes fail by failing to connect, please be patient with us, and know we are only human, but we care, deeply.

Thank you to Vivian Chen for the excellent cover design and illustrations, and Tiffany Barfield for her expert photography.

About the Author

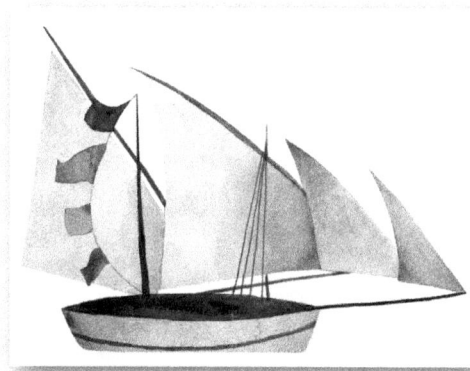

G ary Josephsen, MD, trained at Harbor-UCLA Medical Center. He is a community emergency physician practicing full-time clinical medicine. He also serves as an affiliate professor with Oregon Health Sciences University, teaching physician assistant students in his community ED. Gary lives in Oregon with his wife and two boys. They spend their days playing in the woods while it rains.

www.ingramcontent.com/pod-product-compliance
Lightning Source LLC
Chambersburg PA
CBHW070355200326
41518CB00012B/2239